"... a nurse in the Columbine, Colorado, school district describes responding to the high school on the day of the student shooting..."

—Lisa Romeo,
ForeWord Reviews
Clarion Review

"School nurses are responsible for the health of thousands of students, and do more than simply dispense daily medications and apply Band-Aids."

—Kirkus Reviews

"... with the changing economy, school nurses have become the front line of health care... because of recent efforts to keep children with health challenges in the general school population, school nurses have had to step up their game."

—BlueInk Review

"As these stories show, school nurses must be prepared for everything from nosebleeds to cardiac arrests to school shootings."

—Kirkus Reviews

ANGELS IN DISGUISE

ANGELS IN DISGUISE

Stories From America's School Nurses

Compiled and Edited by

Dolores H. McNany, EdD, MA, RN, NJSCSN

iUniverse LLC
Bloomington

Angels in Disguise
Stories From America's School Nurses

Copyright © 2011, 2014 Dolores H. McNany, EdD, MA, RN, NJSCSN

BAND-AID® Brand Adhesive Bandages are registered and licensed exclusively to Johnson & Johnson Consumer Companies, Inc.

Ritalin® is a registered trademark of Novartis Pharmaceuticals Corp. Manufactured for: Alliant Pharmaceuticals, Inc.

iUniverse books may be ordered through booksellers or by contacting:

iUniverse LLC
1663 Liberty Drive
Bloomington, IN 47403
www.iuniverse.com
1-800-Authors (1-800-288-4677)

ISBN: 978-1-4620-0626-7 (sc)
ISBN: 978-1-4620-0627-4 (hc)
ISBN: 978-1-4620-0628-1 (e)

Library of Congress Control Number: 2011904433

Printed in the United States of America

iUniverse rev. date: 01/21/2014

Cover Design and Illustration: Maureen Jansen, BFA
Photographer: Tim McNany, BA

For my husband, five children,
and seven grandchildren, with love

Contents

Foreword.. xv

Preface.. xvii

Acknowledgments xxi

First Response   1

Nurse to the Playground
Ellen Williams, MEd, BSN, RN 2
My Small Life
Tamara J. Smylie, BS, RN, NCSN 3
One Toe on the Gas
Alexis J. Strickland, RN 5
We Were All Columbine
Elizabeth (Betty) Fitzpatrick, MS, SNP, RN 8

Front Line   11

More than Frostbite
Laura Petrowich, BSN, RN 12
From Novice to Mentor with Some Help from My Friends
Heidi Toth, MS, MSN, RN, CIC 15
Appeal to County Commissioners
Julia A. Derouen, MEd, NCC, LPCA 19
Beyond Bandages
Linda Betley, MSN, RN 21
The Many Hats of This Nurse
Barbara L. Filer, BSN, RN, CSN 23
Little Did I Know
Tracy Jones, RN 25
Knock-Knock
Patricia A. DeLorenze, LPN 27
School Nursing in a Rural Community
Anne E. Allen, BSN, RN, OCN 29

Baseline Data   31

Waiting To Be Bored
Kathleen M. Halkins, BSN, RN 32
3,659 and Counting
Carol Ann Scalgione, RN 35
No Monotony Here
Jeanmarie Ringwood, MA, RN, CSN 37
From 7:00 a.m. to 3:30 p.m.
Laurie Feldkamp, BSN, RN 38
Back and Forth Between Schools
Sherri Verdun, BS, RN, CSN 41
Big Luxuries in a Little Town
Candi Thomas, BSN, RN 43
A Day in the Life of a School Nurse
Phyllis Gentry, RN 46
The Hardest Job I Have Ever Loved
Amy Jayne Barnes, MA, BSN, RN 48
School Nursing Versus Fear of Working Nights
Renie Sullivan, MEd, BSN, RN 53
Do Vegetarians Eat Animal Crackers?
Lori E. Robson, BSN, RN, CSN 55

Critical Care   58

It Mattered to This One
Shirley Rodriguez, BSN, RN, CSNP 59
Here's the Deal
Kayla Mohling, BSN, RN 61

Triage   64

You Did What?
Tamara Dorsett, BSN, RN 65
More Than Twenty Cents per Student
Donna C. Maginness, BSN, RN 67
Everything Hurts
Laura D. Fell, BSN, RN 70
Between Filling Out Reports
Ruthann Hatt, BSN, RN 71
One Child at a Time
Sunny Kirkham, RN 73

"Tell Me ... I Can Take It!"
Shirley Rodriguez, BSN, RN, CSNP 76

Counseling 78

Special Passes
Wanda Bouvier, RNC 79
Super Solution
Patricia Marsh-Thorell, BSN, RN 81
The Stomachache
Gloria Jean Reynolds, BSN, RN, CSN 83
Everything Isn't Always What I Hear
Patti J. Twaddle, RN 84
The Little Boy and His Shoes
Gloria Jean Reynolds, BSN, RN, CSN 85
Yes, the Nurse Is Here ... You're Looking at Him
Robert D. Naugle, AND, BFA 86
A Mighty Purpose
Laurie Rufolo, MSN, RN 89
The Proper Care and Feeding of a School Nurse
Patricia H. Allocca, LCSW, RN, CSN 91

Evaluation 93

A "Plum" of a Job
Nina R. Fekaris, MS, BSN, RN, NCSN 94
Every Student Deserves a School Nurse
Verna Thompson, BSN, RN 96
Outside the Gym Closet
Dorothy Patrock, MS, RN, SANE-A 98
Grateful to Serve
Carol Ray, LPN 100
The Acorn and the Tree
Eunice Arendt, RN 101
Swine Flu
Beth H. Wipf, BSN, RN 103

Multitasking 105

Perfecting the Art of Multitasking
Julie Parker, RN 106

Just in Time
Melanie Sharpton, RN 108
Phone Calls to E-mail
Janne M. DeMarco, MS, BS, RN, LPN, CSN 110
Who Am I and What Hat Should I Wear Today?
Marcia Howard, BSN, RN, PHN 111

Intervention   112

Substitute Mom
Marilyn L. Hebert, BS, RN 113
School Nurses Are Public Health Allies
Wendy Doremus, MS, RN, NP-BC 116
Ponytail Lesson
Phyllis E. Kobayashi, School Health Aide 118
Together We Can Make a Difference to a Child
Rosamarie Cruz, MEd, BSN, RN, CSN 120
From Head Lice to Budget Cuts
Mary A. O'Neill, MA, RN, CSN 121
It's the Little Things That Count
Sharon L. King, RN, NCSN 123
First Year
Domichellei Walker, RN 124
Lessons Learned
Robin Halemeyer, BSN, RN, CSN 125
A Piece of My Heart
Vici McClure, BSN, RN 126
The Eighth-Grade Graduation
Robin Halemeyer, BSN, RN, CSN 129
The Blue Denim Hat
Jean Anne Kamrath, MSFL, BSN, RN 131

Contributors 133

Foreword

In this compilation of letters from school nurses, Dolores H. McNany, EdD, MA, RN, NJSCSN, gathered, after nearly three years of persistent pursuit of school nurses throughout the nation, insights from the experts. This book is a snapshot of the character that makes a school nurse so unique to her geographic location but so similar to the caregivers of schoolchildren throughout our country.

You will discover the heart, body, and soul of dedicated, committed nurses upholding the standards and "best practices of school nursing" in every school nurse's office. Whether a school nurse works with a school population of one school with two hundred fifty students or four schools with eight thousand students and takes her "office in a bag" with "one toe on the gas," a practice one nurse in Michigan describes as "drive-by school nursing," she will provide the same high quality of nursing care to each child.

Regardless of a state's nurse-to-student ratio practices, these school nurses provide the "gold standard of care" to students and will continue to do so until there is a nurse in every building because they believe, as McNany does, that "Every child deserves access to a school nurse."

As state-mandated and federally mandated programs continue to extract high costs to educate our students, McNany demonstrates that school nurses carry out their professional practice and regard it as the "toughest job they have ever loved." These letters provide the common threads of:

> *Love* ~ one nurse giving money to a child so that she could buy a flower for her mother on Mother's Day,
> *Humor* ~ one child not wanting to eat animal crackers to settle his stomach because he was a vegetarian, and
> *Trauma* ~ school nurses calming students during a lockdown for a "shooter in the school."

This is a different kind of book. The editor's need to have school nurses be heard has driven her to collect the stories to answer the question "What do school nurses do?" and to answer that question in their own words. We extend our gratitude to Dr. McNany for her efforts to obtain these stories detailing the experiences of school nurses and to educate the public regarding the critical position of the school nurse.

Judith A. Woop, MEd, RN, NJSCSN
School Nurse Certification Program Coordinator
Department of Education, Caldwell College, New Jersey
Past President New Jersey State School Nurses Association

Preface

"My mother said, 'Go see the nurse.'"

Throughout my twenty-year career as a school nurse, how often did I hear these words from a child at my office door? The child stood in the doorway with a dirty bandaged finger or a cough, maybe holding back tears or experiencing unfamiliar pain. Many parents who are unable to afford adequate health insurance, or cannot stay at home from work, send their children to school and trust that the school nurse will see to it that their children will get the care they need. Parents expected me, as the school nurse, to administer medical treatment and clinical procedures to their children.

The perception the general public has of the twenty-first-century school nurse is antiquated. The general public knows little about the rich educational, clinical, social, and psychological experience and skills that school nurses possess. With the advancement of medical technology and the inclusion of medically fragile children, school nurses are the professionals who are best prepared to meet the necessary medical and clinical needs of students. Applying Band-Aids to scraped knees, checking for fevers, or taking out splinters are a minuscule part of today's school nursing procedures. Most cases are handled by the school nurse on the spot, with first aid or tender loving care.

For all school nurses, there are those times and incidents that, for different reasons, leave them with deep impressions that they will never forget. As a school nurse, I too experienced, along with parents, both the happy and sad times in a child's life. School nurses are now the frontline primary health care provider for today's students and school personnel. The caseload and complex responsibilities for school nurses have changed from what was at one time considered a "minor health care office" into a full-fledged health clinic.

By sharing my experiences and knowledge with the general public, my goal is to introduce and provide a behind-the-scenes view of how all school nurses meet the daily demands by drawing upon their knowledge, leadership skills, and clinical expertise. People will come to understand and recognize the dedication school nurses have for all children. Underlying and woven within each story is the often unrecognized yet endless energy school nurses possess as they care for our schoolchildren while juggling a myriad of tasks set forth by school districts and state and federal laws. The role of the school nurse is complex, and it is exactly these complexities that need to be revealed to the public sector in order to gain their confidence and understanding regarding the importance of the role that school nurses play in the lives of their children.

School nursing is a specialized branch of professional nursing within the field of nursing. School nurses come from diverse backgrounds, training, education, and experiences. They draw upon their medical knowledge and clinical expertise to recognize and respond to mental, emotional, and physical needs of children at all levels of wellness or illness. Holistic care of the child from head to toe is the utmost important part of their daily life.

In the medical office each day, often unnoticed in the bustle of a school day, the school nurse demonstrates strong, loving, and compassionate care for the children. School nurses have the highest privilege and honor and the greatest responsibility: that of teaching and molding young healthy hearts and minds, healthy bodies, and healthy lifestyles. Each day, school nurses across America make a difference in children's lives and help prepare them to become healthy, responsible, and productive members of society. The most rewarding endeavor for a school nurse is to see each and every child reach their full potential, mentally and physically. School nurses deserve recognition and should be applauded for their devotion to children, yet sadly, the school nurse is seldom in the limelight.

My intent for this book of collective stories is to enlighten and stimulate the reader's mind to appreciate the devotion of school nurses, as told through their personal stories. Unfortunately, many school nurses in this country are responsible for more than two thousand to three thousand students in attendance at two to five schools (or more), regardless of the health of the student population. Regardless of the total number of students, each child will receive the same devotion to the best of the school nurse's abilities.

The health of the school population served by school nurses today includes, but is not limited to, services performed, such as: counseling, social work, serving as a resource person, monitoring health records, and providing medical assessments through individualized health care management plans. Physical ailments presented by students, to name only a few, include: seizures, obesity, bipolar disorder, depression, pregnancy, ADHD, life-threatening allergies, catheterizations, and screening programs, with written referrals for follow-up notification on all medical and physical ailments. Moreover, the responsibility of training unlicensed personnel to assist the school nurse and health concerns of the school employees, administrators, and even parents have been incorporated into the school nurses' increased responsibilities. In addition, concerns regarding school laws, state and federal mandates, plans as first responders in school shootings and terrorist attacks, the Nurse Practice Act, and legal issues in school health services definitely demonstrate that the "plate is full" for all school nurses across the country. The successful delivery of school health services depends upon the ability of the school nurse to reach out to parents in the community and convince them that she or he is an advocate for their children.

School nurses are an integral part of the school system, with a direct bearing upon the wellness and educational outcome of the student. If a child is not feeling well, he or she cannot mentally or physically concentrate on learning in the classroom. Parents whose children come under the care of school nurses find it difficult to understand the limitations and standards set by districts and state and federal laws that school nurses are required to uphold. Additionally, the book will help parents and others to understand how difficult it is for the school nurse to accomplish all that is required of her. Misconceptions by school personnel and school administrators regarding the role of the school nurse in an educational setting leave the school nurse with a feeling of isolation.

To add to the dilemma, school nursing positions are being threatened by budgetary crises facing school districts all across the United States. The position of the school nurse should not be subject to budget reduction. Many states lack mandated laws regarding the hiring of school nurses. Instead, they rely on recommended guidelines proposed by the federal government. Parents are often understandably confused by limitations and standards set by state and federal law. If school nurses are to be successful in providing high-quality health services to the children in their school systems and under their care, parental support is vital. School nursing associations, school nurse leaders at state, county, and local levels, and school nurses themselves must be ever vigilant in taking a proactive approach with legislators at all levels of government. Our most precious commodity, the youth of this nation, will be the ones most affected by the decision to cut back on school nurse positions. Additionally, it is my goal that this information enlighten parents, teachers, principals, school administrators, and state legislators to recognize the invaluable services that school nurses provide in enabling every child to fulfill his or her potential.

Regardless of the state or its location in our nation, I found through personal contact and telephone conversations with countless school nurses that they are universally dedicated to caring for the mental and physical well-being of the children in their care. School nurses are dedicated to helping children realize their full potential: intellectually, emotionally, and physically.

School nurses have many wonderful stories to tell, stories that can help others better understand and appreciate their vital role in our schools and communities. Perhaps these stories from school nurses across America, in their very spirited and personal anecdotes, will enlighten everyone about the reservoirs of health care available to our school children.

I believe other school nurses will thoroughly enjoy reading their fellow school nurses' stories and recognize themselves and their own commitment to serving children each day with devotion. I firmly believe that parents after reading the book will have a better understanding of the role of the school nurse and, equipped with new knowledge, will support the school nurse, including advocating for the hiring of a school nurse for every school facility in their community.

For twenty years, I worked and taught as a school nurse/health education teacher in both public and private schools and was the watch guard of children's physical, mental, and healthy lifestyle at all levels of wellness and illness. I counseled parents, children, and school staff on the importance of maintaining a healthy lifestyle in order for children to become productive members of society. I feel blessed by having shared in those events, most sweet to most painful, and know that this is a sentiment experienced by every school nurse. These memories are with me forever, as those of my nurse colleagues are with them. I am forever grateful for being part of such a wonderful profession.

Dolores H. McNany, EdD, MA, RN, NJSCSN
Assistant Director Emeritus
School Nurse/Health Teacher Certification Program
Department of Education, Caldwell College, Caldwell, New Jersey
Editor

Acknowledgments

The research to complete this book was several years in the making. Without support from school nurses across America, I would not have been able to tell, in their own words, their stories about school nursing. Eagerly, they submitted their stories and took time out of their busy lives to express their personal feelings regarding the difficulties they faced each and every day caring for schoolchildren. I am astonished by their willingness and openness to talk to me about their need to have someone listen and champion their cause. I am honored.

During the research, many wonderful stories were sent to me by the school nurses; unfortunately, numerous stories were edited or eliminated in order to contain only the core facts and to protect confidentiality. I still feel sad about this, mostly because every school nurse put so much time and heart into writing their stories; some of you will be disappointed, and I ask for your understanding regarding the necessity of editorial revisions.

My wholehearted thank you goes out to all the school nurses who supported my goal to have this book published. Fortunately, more and more men each year join the school nursing profession. The choice to use the pronoun "she" when referring to school nurses in this book is an editorial preference and not in any way meant to disregard or diminish the professionalism, dedication, and commitment of male school nurses. This book provides a venue for all school nurses to share our collective stories, a venue where our voices can be heard.

I acknowledge the encouragement, personal advice, and information from my many friends and colleagues, who graciously provided a steady stream of enthusiasm throughout the duration of the research to the formulating of the book. I also thank my dear friend Richard Thayer, PhD, for his advice and encouragement. I extend my sincere appreciation to all those at iUniverse, who assisted and encouraged me through numerous editing stages and for publishing these heartwarming stories.

I am most grateful and express my love to my family for believing in me. To my son Tim for taking professional photographs and to son-in-law Harry for helping me when I could not figure out how to correct the mistakes I made on my computer. To my daughter Maureen for creating the cover design/illustration and for her technical knowledge in formatting the book and editing assistance; and son-in-law Lou, who introduced me to online publishing, I am very grateful. The continual encouragement received from my daughter Colleen, my sons Danny and Gene, and Gene's wife, my daughter-in-law Kristin, is extremely meaningful. A special thank you I extend to my husband Eugene, who helped me stuff and stamp one thousand envelopes, carry the boxes to the post office, and encouraged me to continue even when I felt overwhelmed; I am forever thankful for his loving support.

To my typist, Pat, thank you for so graciously giving your time and doing such a wonderful job sorting out deletions and typing the manuscript. To a dear friend and colleague, Judith A. Woop, MEd, RN, NJSCSN, I express my sincere thanks for reviewing this book and for your wonderful words of endorsement in the Foreword. To Sister Mary John Kearney, OP, my mentor and dearest friend, I extend my heartfelt love and gratitude for her constant encouragement to continue writing. Finally, but most importantly, I express my deep appreciation and say thank you to a very dear friend who prefers to remain nameless who helped organize the layout of the book. Without her diligence and creative mind, which provided a constant source of mentoring and assistance with proofreading and computer expertise, this book would remain unfinished.

Dolores H. McNany, EdD, MA, RN, NJSCSN

First Response

Whether a child is lying on the playground unconscious, a teacher is holding the tip of a cut-off finger, or there's been a shooting inside the school building, the school nurse must be prepared to face any and all challenges. When you investigate these stories, you will come to know the love and devotion these courageous school nurses have in order to "act under fire."

NURSE TO THE PLAYGROUND

It was a beautiful day. Autumn, with all the feel of the change from summer to fall, was in the air. The day felt different because it was the first day of the new district trial of half-day classes, with professional development in the afternoon. The office staff and I were chattering away when the call came over the radio from the PE coach: "I need the nurse to the playground!" Now, this is not an unusual event, and I typically return the call with, "What do I need to bring?" My question was interrupted with a frantic, "She's not breathing!"

Knowing the coach as I did and hearing the tone of his voice, I immediately started running to the playground. The principal was close behind. As I ran through the halls, I radioed the office to activate Emergency Medical Services (EMS). When I ran out the door to the playground, I saw in the far soccer field that the coach was bent over a student lying on the ground.

When I got to them, the coach stated that he thought the student was breathing after all. A quick assessment found agonal breaths and no pulse. I immediately started CPR and asked the coach if he knew how to help. He started the chest compressions, and I continued breaths. We continued full CPR until the EMS arrived nine minutes later and took over.

After three shocks with a defibrillator and an IV line in place, EMS requested that I continue with compressions. After one more minute of compressions and breaths via an ambubag, one of the greatest moments in my nursing career occurred. The student took an unassisted breath while my hands were still on her chest.

Certainly not all encounters school nurses have with students are of this gravity, and if they are, not all have positive outcomes. However, the presence of nurses in the schools makes other important differences in the lives of students and their families on a daily basis.

Ellen Williams, MEd, BSN, RN
New Mexico

My Small Life

I live a small, quiet life. Every day is pretty much the same as the one before it—lots of bandages, cough drops, and hugs. You try to feel out the ones that need a break from the tedium of school, the kids that just need a few minutes of sanctuary on the cot in the back. These kids, no matter what the age, are sometimes hard to differentiate from those with real stomachaches. Usually you can see it in their eyes.

The event that changed my life happened during my first or second year as a school nurse, after twenty years of hospital shifts and home health patients. I finally found my niche, and I felt incredibly lucky. How many people really ever love their jobs? I mean love it every single day? I was so very thankful for my small, happy life.

My assignment was to cover a middle school while the regular school nurse was away having her knee replaced. It was Friday, the end to a fun week, the last before Christmas vacation. The doors in the hallways still had shreds of crepe paper and glitter from the winter door contest. Teachers were smiling, and the kids were high on sugar from their parties. After a long afternoon of headaches and stomachaches from too much soda and cookies, I was ready to go home and enjoy the holidays. At around three o'clock, I began the ritual of double-checking the lock on the med cabinet, putting away the scissors and antibiotic ointment, and charting the last of the students I'd treated.

I hear yelling in the hallway outside the nurse's office, and here come a couple of sixth graders, trying to spit out a few words in between gasps of air. Something about a kid falling on the track and a bloody nose? "Why don't you have him come in here?" I ask. "After all, everything I need is here in the office, not out there on the track." "No, no, you have to come out; a student is hurt, and the teacher wants you to come."

I grab the field trip pack and start out to the athletic field, following the sixth graders who came to fetch me. It's quite a jog out to the track, through the building, the commons, and past the gym. As I reach a point where I can see more clearly, I see a small figure lying on the track, with many confused, young faces huddled around him. Then I start running. Many of you know the feeling I am about to describe. The moment when the whole world stops, and all you can hear is your own heart beating, your own breathing, and you feel as though someone has pushed you off of a tall building—that queasy feeling deep inside. It looked as if he had just fallen face down in the gravel, unable to break his fall, not a moment to react.

I can remember screaming at the bewildered PE teacher to please get all the other students inside the gym, barking orders to another teacher to call 911 and then call the student's parents.

Smell and taste can bring back some of the most powerful memories. Have you ever noticed that? A whiff of someone's perfume or skin cream can elicit fond memories of loved ones and of the past. After giving rescue breathing and CPR, I can still taste the minty gum he was chewing that afternoon. I can feel the gravel digging into my knees, and I can see my tears dropping onto the front of his shirt, staining it with dark circles as I am doing chest compressions. The ambulance came. How I hated telling the parents to meet me at the hospital, knowing that their child may already have passed away. I was overwhelmed by this tragic event despite the words of hope and optimism voiced by teachers and staff.

I tried to find some shred of reason for this death, or more selfishly, a reason why I was there that day instead of someone else. Was I fast enough? Smart enough? Brave enough? Why me instead of the school's regular nurse?

Then I think of that nurse, bending down on her painfully arthritic knees in the gravel to administer CPR. Trying to run out to the field, running back and forth making phone calls, herding crowds. Maybe I was there that day for a reason. Not a heroic reason, perhaps just a practical one; a reason that involved stronger knees and younger legs. If that's the case, then I can accept that.

As I get older, I think about that day on the track field giving CPR and the sorrow I experienced when this young, precious life passed away. What a life-changing experience it was for me.

This is the first time I have written his story down. Dear boy, you changed me and my small, quiet life.

Tamara J. Smylie, BS, RN, NCSN
New Mexico

One Toe on the Gas

I have worked as a school nurse since November 1982. My situation is somewhat different than what is considered a "normal" school nurse role, as I am in a vocational-technical setting and also have special needs students in a second building. Most of my time is spent with vocational students, primarily juniors and seniors in high school. It can be a challenge trying to decide who is really sick and who just does not want to be here today. There are no sports physicals here or immunization clinic. There is a rocking chair in my room that has been put to so much use I am surprised that it has not had to be replaced.

When I am not sure about whether a student is really sick or has just had a bad day, it helps to put them in the chair and just let them sit a few minutes. As the chair starts to move, they seem to calm down; and many times with no prompting, the story comes out: a fight with parents or boyfriends, concern for a friend who is making bad choices, or problems at work (and it is amazing how many of these kids are working at least twenty hours a week while they try to balance academic needs!). Sometimes a more serious problem will arise with abuse and teen pregnancies.

I am blessed with a great support system here, including a social worker who is always available for the students. Our faculty is also unique. The majority are tradespeople who have gone on to get a teaching degree. They bring years of experience in balancing home and work. I have seen teachers go out to homes to visit students and parents, encouraging and doing whatever it takes to keep the kids in school and on track.

My baptism of fire occurred on my first day at work. I was called to go to the agricultural mechanic's classroom for a teacher who had cut off part of his finger. I did not even know where the room was, so a secretary took me to the classroom. The teacher was at least six feet tall. (I am five feet on a good day with the right shoes.) He was pacing the room with his hands in the air, holding pressure on the injured finger. He said, "Okay, let's get going—you can drive my car; we have to get back before the students get here."

I asked if I could see what he had done, and he said, "I got my hand too close to the exhaust fan, and it pulled me in. It took off the end of my finger."

He never lowered his hands for me to see. I asked him where the fingertip was, and he told me not to worry about it. When I insisted they would want it at the hospital, he gestured in several places and stated, "It's there and there and there—let's go!" We told him he should go by ambulance, and he said,

"There isn't any time for that"; he had to be back by the time the students got there. "We will take my car—it's outside the shop."

I looked at the secretary, and she shrugged her shoulders and said she would let the principal know where we were. We went out the door and to his car. (It looked big enough to be a bus to me). As the secretary helped me in, I asked her to call the hospital to say we were on the way. I got into the car and—surprise, surprise—the seat did not adjust! I had to drive with one toe on the gas and prop myself forward with one hand so I could reach the steering wheel.

We ended up in a backlog of patients ahead of us; and after about two hours, the principal of the school showed up to bring me back. The teacher was still not seen, but they decided that since his car was there, he would come back by himself after he was treated. When I got out to the principal's vehicle, it was a World War II jeep, with canvas covers. Remember, I started in November and was just hustled from the office to the shop, to the car, to the hospital, to the jeep. My coat was still back at work. After I managed to climb in, there was no seat belt and no heat. I did have a little handle on the dash that I could hold onto to keep some balance. I sure needed it. My boss drove like he thought there were land mines all over the road and possibly a tank chasing us.

When I got home that night, I burst into tears. What had I gotten myself into now? But I went back the next day, and I am still here. I decided that if I could make it through that day, there couldn't be much left to surprise me.

Most of the student injuries are minor cuts, burns, bruises, or scrapes as the students become acclimated to the machinery and equipment in their settings. There are some exceptions to this. I have sent students to the hospital (thankfully only five minutes away) with French knife cuts as they learned to slice and dice food. There have been two students who did a marvelous job setting their pants on fire as they were welding. A student in our graphics department thought he could reach the paper in the press before the press got it. When the press was shut down and he was extricated, we had some pretty flat fingers that thankfully were intact. He did regain full use in a few months.

The students with special needs are my favorites. The sheer joy and exuberance they display with the talents they have been given are a humbling experience. In spite of—or possibly because of—their "handicaps," they show a remarkable outlook on life. The love that flows from them is so soothing. We have had tube feedings, catheterizations, dressing changes, splints, and colostomy bags, just to name a few treatments they require. They are the first to smile and say hello, and the last to criticize anyone. Perhaps we could take a lesson from them.

I plan to retire soon. Things have changed so much since I started. While my coworkers are wonderful and appreciative, the rules and regulations have become more than I care to deal with. We have lost the ability to be a part of our children's lives. For those of you who have done this as long as I have, do you remember calling a parent and telling them that Johnny has a headache and asking them if they want you to give him something for the headache? Their word was good enough. Now there are forms for everything. Do you sometimes wonder if you are a secretary or a nurse? Remember taking time to visit families and doing health teaching when it was necessary?

We are going too fast, too eager to get somewhere, but none of us really knows where. It is time for this dinosaur to retire and rest and for the new speedy spaceagers to buzz on in my place. I leave with wonderful memories and no regrets.

Alexis J. Strickland, RN
New York

WE WERE ALL COLUMBINE

I was at work one day, and my superintendent called and said I had to go to Columbine High School immediately. "Something major is going on, and students are trapped in the school." I grabbed my cell phone and headed there. Columbine was one of eighteen high schools in our district. They had an enrollment of two thousand students, were located in an affluent part of the county, and had a reputation of being both academically and athletically successful. Filled with apprehension, I arrived there a little after eleven thirty, with my car radio full of reports of an active shooting in progress. I was not to return home until 1:00 a.m. later that night.

As I arrived on the scene, I was stopped by a police officer who let me in as I showed my ID and told him I was directed there to assist with "crisis response." It was a chaotic scene, with multiple law enforcement personnel arriving, ambulances screeching in, National Guard unloading weapons and vests, and media setting up communication. Within minutes, it was gridlock, with parents coming to add to the confusion and hysteria. Disbelief permeated the scene.

Immediately, police cordoned off the area, and I met with the assistant superintendent and started planning. I had done an all-call to our crisis teams and asked them to respond to the scene. Some got there, and some did not. Shooting was going on inside the building, fire alarms were going off, sprinkler systems were on throughout the school, and we started receiving calls from inside the building where students were trapped. They had TVs on and were watching the rescue efforts outside.

Slowly pieces of information came out to us. We knew there were bodies inside the library. We knew there was a teacher hunkered down in a classroom, bleeding to death. We did not know who, how many, or where the shooters were. Police were outside and reluctant to go in. Floor plans were faxed over, but they were the old plans before the remodel. The shooting finally stopped, and the police decided to go in. I knew this was not going to have a good outcome when one of the National Guardsman went inside the building, came out quickly, and vomited in the bushes.

We set up triage areas. The police escorted trapped students out of the building. They took short statements from them and sent them over to our quickly assembled teams of nurses, social workers, and school psychologists. We gave them emotional support, allowed them to tell us what they saw and experienced, and put them in touch with their loved ones. They were frightened and upset. Most were crying, and some were in shocked silence. All of them had terrible stories to tell. That was when we knew the shooters were indeed students at the high school. We could have never imagined something like this happening in our schools!

We called for school buses to transport these students to a reunification site (the nearest elementary school) where we had directed parents. By the end of the night, the parents remaining at the reunification site were those who had not found their sons or daughters. They looked around, and we looked around. It became clear that they were the ones whose students were never to come home again.

Then we began the long process of planning, reacting, supporting, and trying to make some sense out of the senseless. We had to take care of the victims' families, the physically injured students, and the emotionally traumatized student body, staff, and community, who were reeling from the events of the day. We provided services and support that would go on for years.

The school was a crime site and thus was closed off until the investigation was complete. We had to establish a school site for the Columbine students to finish the school year. We were advised to return to normalcy as quickly as possible. But "normal" would never be the same again.

This seminal event changed forever how schools would respond to an emergency. Emergencies became something more than fire drills and bomb scares. Who ever would have guessed? Immediately, law enforcement became partners with schools, keeping floor plans of schools on CDs in their squad cars. They actually practiced drills with school staff. Communities developed sophisticated emergency response teams. Posttraumatic stress disorder became a commonly understood term. A place called school would never be the same.

And school nurses became leaders for emergency response. They became the drivers of how each school responded and the caretakers in the aftermath of tragedy. They were the consistent experts who were available to students and staff alike. They managed physical symptoms and supported the emotional scars that were carried within the students, not only at Columbine High School but also within all one hundred fifty of our schools. We were "all Columbine." The media coverage was relentless and served to repeatedly traumatize our students and staff.

But never was I more proud of my school nursing staff as they served long hours—without complaining—to support students, staff, families, and community alike. They used all of their many skills to emerge as respected role models for school nurses across the country.

School nursing has changed exponentially since I began my career. The discipline of school nursing has evolved to a complex practice area that requires nurses to be knowledgeable at so many levels. What remains unchanged are the dedication, compassion, flexibility, and ability of the women and men who serve in this field. I am so proud to be one of many who serve our millions of schoolchildren across the United States. What a privilege!

Elizabeth (Betty) Fitzpatrick, MS, SNP, RN
Colorado

Front Line

Keeping students safe from frostbite or using flashlights or miner's headlamps during three months of winter darkness to avoid accidents are another facet of school nursing. School nurses wear many hats during their daily care of schoolchildren and still manage to meet an abundance of challenges brought to their "doorstep." From wet pants to Band-Aids, immunization shots to telling jokes to alleviate a child's fear—the further you read, the more you will recognize how different but equal school nurses are in performing their duties.

More than Frostbite

School nursing is more than frostbite in Alaska. The students go outside for recess until the thermometer plummets to twenty degrees below zero. There are seldom any school days missed due to cold weather or snow. It would have to be close to fifty below zero before parents start listening for school closures on the radio.

Parents safeguard their elementary students from the cold by layering them each with a hat, parka, snow pants, neck gaiter, mittens, and boots. If they have a kindergartener, putting on the gear is typically a fifteen-minute process before the bus arrives. Parents will routinely stuff extra socks in a backpack to use in case a mitten is lost or for an extra layer on the children's feet at recess.

Parents also protect their students by making sure that they are seen in the twenty-two hours of winter darkness by giving them miners' headlamps or flashlights to carry while waiting for the bus. The students also have reflective tape that is sewn onto their backpacks and jackets. The local Parent Teacher Associations provide this service by having a group of volunteers with sewing machines spend a week in the school applying reflective tape to winter gear.

I am the school nurse who watches the students waddle off the buses and past my office each day. They look like colorful marshmallows bumping off each other on their way to class. Their gear can range from handmade fur hats to fuchsia fleece caps. The coats run the gamut from Columbia outdoor garments to handmade fur-trimmed parkas. As far as the mittens go, I just look to see that they have two.

My busy time for triaging students occurs during recess. Our playground has a man-made sledding hill and an ice rink. The students are allowed to bring their own sleds and skates to school. I also have a sled that I use, rather than a wheelchair, to retrieve someone with a twisted ankle from the slide. The slide is a popular attraction if there is still frost clinging to it. The surface propels the rider beyond the normal landing zone and into my office for ice rash. As funny as it sounds, I treat it with more ice.

A good recess is measured by how many ice packs I hand out. The record in my office is eighteen packs. That was a chaotic day. I had five students present with bee stings simultaneously, and they had multiple bites. I gave out Benadryl by the capful and lined them up on the cot to face me so that I could watch for an anaphylactic reaction and treat other bumps and cuts at the same time. Thankfully, none of them had difficulty breathing. The

Benadryl made them sleepy for the afternoon, which was not a bad thing, according to one teacher.

I suffered from an adrenaline rush that I was told would not happen as a school nurse. I cannot remember which hospital nurse told me that, but I would like for her to take on the care plans of five hundred students and recall which ones are allergic to bee stings.

The sight of blood is common in my sink due to nosebleeds from the dry, cold air. Normally the scarf the student is wearing will help stop the deluge. I use a stain stick on the scarf and gauze on the student. It usually stops bleeding when a bit of pressure is applied. Blood also comes from the one day each year that one kindergartener dares another one to stick their tongues on playground equipment at twenty below zero. It sets up a chain reaction of about four to six students that need help. The playground attendant carries a water flask in his shirt pocket for just such an occasion. Some get scared and lose a few taste buds when they rip it off. Others will wait for the warm water to release them. By the time they see me, I tell them that a bandage will not stick to their tongue and send them to class. They never repeat the experience again.

Another common ailment is splinters from the birch and spruce trees that surround the playground. For thirty minutes every day, the area is transformed into fairy houses and forts. I hold an oversize magnifying glass, while the student uses the tweezers. Their eyesight is better than mine, so it saves time hunting for the painful culprit.

The playground takes on different safety obstacles due to the weather. The students wear mittens when navigating the monkey bars during the winter and come into my office during warm weather to complain about blisters across the palms of their hands. I challenge them to figure out what is different between summer and winter when they twist their hands on the monkey bars. They feel like detectives when they solve the problem.

The swings also take on different safety problems in the winter. The snow packs underneath the swings so the students bend their knees outward so they will not hit the snow as they glide back and forth. The distance between the swing and the landing zone is shorter during the winter. They forget to compensate for the distance when the snow melts when dismounting the swing. Their knees buckle, and they tumble face forward in the mud and water holes during "Breakup."

Breakup is a special time on the playground because the students are allowed to take their coats off when it becomes fifty degrees, and they run through the water holes with rubber boots on. It is also the time of year that the lost and found pile grows by the day because the snowmelt reveals jackets that were left on the playground in October. I spend triage time looking for clothing that might fit to warm up a mud-soaked student.

I do see the occasional student that has frostbite. The treatment is simple. Be gentle and kind to the skin. Place warm hands on top of cold cheeks or fingers and thaw. If they are able to smile and hold your hand, they are ready to go back to class. All of my students are able to hold number two yellow pencils and smile at me in the hall, so my plan of care to keep them safe until they see their parents again must be working.

Laura Petrowich, BSN, RN
Alaska

From Novice to Mentor with Some Help from My Friends

What is a school nurse? I never even considered it for a possible career until I was finishing my bachelor's degree and had the opportunity to visit a school to see what school nursing was all about. Little did I know at that time that I would end up choosing school nursing as my passion. When the idea of a school nurse career piqued my interest after having my second daughter, I enrolled in courses for my school nurse certificate. It would be a job that worked well for my family, with summers off to enjoy my favorite place, the beach. The next thing I did was join my county school nurse association so I could learn more about this career and start networking. I finished up my certificate and took my first job, covering two schools a half mile apart, and joined our state and national school nurses' associations.

As all school nurses learn, getting that certificate is like first getting your nursing license. It is the tip of the iceberg, and you find out you only know the basics: screenings, Band-Aids, and health education. At the time of my first job, in most health offices, there were no e-mail and Internet access, let alone a computer. We did not even have a district directory, and I had no idea who the other nurses were in the district. Midway through my year of covering two schools, they moved me to the high school when the nurse there retired. Okay, I could do this new job, I thought.

We had frozen weather, and they had to close the schools for a week. Wow, this is a great career: I get snow days. Isn't that the kind of typical comment we hear from others when they learn we work in a school? How naïve I was! By May, I had my first student come to me because she was pregnant and needed help. Isn't that what we have guidance counselors for? No, they said, "That's your job." Thankfully I had my professional organizations, where I had already started networking and developing those relationships with other school nurses that helped me through. I found a great mentor and other colleagues as I stumbled through that job crisis.

By the time I moved on to another high school, my counseling skills with pregnant teens were good, and I even started a support group. I enjoyed a burst of confidence in my career choice! However, reality set in, and working in a high school with adolescents today sure teaches you a lot. I quickly realized I still had a lot to learn as I looked to my nurse colleagues to assist me with dealing with attempted suicide, substance abuse, gender issues, death of a staff member, practice of witchcraft and animal sacrifice, and diet pill abuse. And, of course, there were the dreaded sports physicals. Everyone else told me how easy this job must be and how it must be stress free!

At the time, I did not have an outside phone line, and we had to use the switchboard operator to make a call. Things were going well. The administration had promised me a computer and I really enjoyed working with the students, but I still wanted my own phone line. I was also working at the local community hospital and had just completed my advanced cardiac life support course. Good thing, because soon after, a twelfth grader came in to my health office saying she did not feel too good—and she definitely did not look too good. You know how school nurses need to develop those rapid assessment skills?

"Okay, come sit down and talk to me," I said. I listened to her heart—oh, really rapid heart rate. I calmly asked, "Are you taking anything?" Meanwhile, all the differential diagnoses ran through my head as I told the student to lie down on the cot so I could get a blood pressure reading. It was very low, and her heart rate was still rapid, her color pale. This was not good. I calmly called 911, and the paramedics were there in an instant. Thankfully, because she was unconscious by then; and when they put her on the cardiac monitor, she was in an unstable ventricular tachycardia.

The paramedics tried to use their cellular phone inside my office; this was in the dark ages before the common use of cell phones and cell towers. They could not get through for medical orders. "Okay, let's use your phone," they said, but remember, I said calls had to go through the school switchboard. The operator was arguing with me that she could not disconnect someone else's call. That did not go over too well with me.

Finally the paramedics were able to get through and received orders to give my student intravenous adenosine, which causes a systole before it works. Here I am in my school nurse office with my student, and we are in the midst of a code. I thought that only happened at the hospital. The student was stabilized to a sinus rhythm and transferred to the hospital, where they diagnosed her with a cardiac condition that was successfully treated with a cardiac ablation. She came back to school a few days later and thanked me for saving her life.

I still wanted my phone line. As nurses in the education field, we know how tough it is to get even those seemingly simple things and I had to seize the moment. I tactfully wrote up the incident and gave it to my administrator, and the nurse's office finally got that outside phone line.

While I loved the high school, I wanted to move to a district that had more choices and more school nurses. This was a one-school district with over one thousand students, and it was lonely to practice in isolation. An opening came up in another town, and I moved to a middle school with less than five hundred students in a district that had seven other nurses, a procedure manual for school nursing, a phone line, and a computer. I was in heaven and started working on developing my skills with the middle school students. I had recently enrolled in a master's program, was expanding my counseling skills, and kept networking with my colleagues.

There was always so much to learn, and again my school nurse colleagues were always there teaching me. A group of us applied for a grant through the Environmental Protection Agency and went to Washington, DC, together to bring back the Indoor Air Quality Program to other districts. It was time away from families on our own time, but so rewarding to work with other nurses who shared the same philosophy. While in Washington, we visited the Vietnam Memorial with one of our school nurses who had been a nurse in Vietnam. We were all overcome with emotion sharing the moment with her, our school nurse colleague.

The Internet was now available, and I continued to learn new things in regard to school nursing every day of my career. Now I was able to share my knowledge with aspiring school nurses, and I looked for innovative ways to make changes. I love to learn and teach, so I became involved in my school's peer leadership program, and I became the first nurse in my district who was a member of our health curriculum committee. I was fortunate that the school administration was willing to listen and support new ideas.

While my professional life has always been about learning new skills, it still comes down to the human touch. In the past year, my school district has experienced devastating student and staff losses that have impacted each and every one of us. As school nurses, we know we carry those burdens. We counsel staff members through their illnesses, work through losses, and have to keep many things confidential. School nurses cannot talk about our work problems in the lunchroom due to maintaining confidentiality. Some days we feel like we are carrying the world's weight on our shoulders. Day after day and through it all, we must be brave. But remember, we have each other to get through those days. I am always grateful and cherish the friendships I have with my school nurse friends because they understand what it is like to walk in my shoes. Without them, I would not have embraced school nursing as I do.

When I received the state school nurse award, I was humbled because I know I am not any different than each and every one of all the school nurses practicing today. After my county nominated me, I had to organize and write down my accomplishments as part of the process. All school nurses could do the same, and we are all carrying around school nurse stories. Each and every one of the nation's school nurses has saved a life, and every day, very quietly, they make differences in countless lives. Most times our efforts are not formally recognized, so it is up to us to support each other and make changes in our profession.

Above all, we must remember what brought us into the field of school nursing. The only way to be truly satisfied is to believe that what you do is great work and to love what you do. We must be aware of the challenges, the needs, and the opportunities we have before us. Think about our purpose. What is our vision? These are questions we need to ask ourselves. A school nurse is in a position of leadership, and this leadership is cultivated over time. Our goal is to get our vision and purpose across to others and become leaders of our own profession. Do not be trapped in the bureaucracy. Have the courage to follow your own curiosity and intuition. School nurses must stand up for what we believe in and be willing to look beyond and toward the future, while continuing to advocate for and protect the health and safety of our students. Each and every one of us has the ability to determine our own destiny in our school nurse career.

Heidi Toth, MS, MSN, RN, CIC
New Jersey

Appeal to County Commissioners

As a teacher, each day I see the need for more school nurses to serve our students. Teachers are trained and obligated to educate our children. School counselors are trained and obligated to meet social and emotional needs of students. Nowhere in our preparation to be educators were we prepared to meet the medical needs of students. Teachers and staff in our schools spend a significant amount of time each day seeing that students receive proper medical attention for chronic illnesses and accidental injury because we don't have an adequate number of school nurses.

School nurses *could* be a positive influence on our schools and academic achievement, but we are told we don't have funds to create more positions. Research reveals that the presence of a trained school nurse has been shown to increase attendance, test scores, and the graduation rate, all of which are prominent issues. This issue is a priority and must be addressed.

Some nurses serve multiple schools totaling over three thousand students. The national recommended ratio is one nurse for every seven hundred fifty students. That leaves each school with a nurse about one day a week, if no other emergencies arise. In that time, the nurse has to maintain medical records, communicate with parents and staff about cases, provide health education in the classrooms, coordinate vision screenings, and tend to numerous student referrals for multiple medical concerns. The number of students in each school seems to be increasing each year; however, the county has not increased the number of school nurses to compensate for this growth. Currently school nurses are overtaxed and stretched past their ability to attend to the number of medical cases.

Today, more than ever before, there is a need for school nurses. The No Child Left Behind and Individuals with Disabilities Education Act legislations force schools to ensure that all students receive an education. These types of legislation are holding counties accountable for providing the services to meet the needs of all students, including those with medical conditions.

Many times, teachers and staff feel inadequate and vulnerable assisting students with medical conditions. The Care for Children with Diabetes legislation now mandates that each school train two people to tend to the medical needs of students with diabetes. This includes testing their blood sugar, injecting insulin shots, operating insulin pumps, and giving glucagon shots when there's a rapid low blood sugar. This involves the potential to come in contact with blood-borne pathogens, as well as greatly affect the health of a child.

Teachers are concerned that they will be held liable for error and feel uncomfortable in providing such services. The funds to staff more nurses to better respond to these cases would be far less than the cost of a lawsuit against a school system for not providing care or providing care that was not by a properly trained professional. It is essential that we keep children who have chronic health problems in school, but it is also essential that we provide school nurses so our teachers can *teach*. The state academic curriculum becomes more rigorous each year, and we are still adding to the responsibilities that teachers have. Providing medical treatment during a lesson should not be asked of our teaching staff.

The diverse population makes for an especially compelling argument for school nurses. Many students do not have or cannot afford to go to the doctor. In many cases, it is the school nurse that identifies the need for medical treatment and can advocate for our students.

School nurses are a valuable resource in our schools. They provide counsel and medical assistance for all incidents from small scrapes to life-threatening emergencies. If we are able to provide a safe and nurturing environment for our students and ensure that they are well nourished and healthy, they have a better chance of achieving their greatest potential. Currently, many of my students are concerned with abuse, parents and siblings who use drugs, when they will eat next, and where they will clean themselves. All of these issues call for the proper medical attention and counseling that only trained professional nurses and counselors can provide.

What makes me the most upset is to see a child who is physically in pain or struggling with a chronic condition who is told, "The school nurse is not here today." We should not be telling our children to wait. When we tell them to wait, when their needs are not being met, we are telling them we don't care, they are not important, and we don't have time for them.

Issues that I have seen have included chronic lice infestation due to insanitary living conditions, malnutrition, asthma, severe allergies, seizures, heart conditions, behavior and emotional disorders that require medication, laryngospasms, and fragile diabetes. All of these cases require daily medical attention. The majority of the week, teachers and staff take time out of their schedules to assist students. What results is a lack of supervision of the remaining students, as well as lost academic time. The need for more sophisticated medical monitoring in the school setting must be addressed by our school district. If we fail to provide an adequate nursing staff, we risk failing our students. That's not a risk I want to take.

Julia A. Derouen, MEd, NCC, LPCA
North Carolina

Beyond Bandages

The role of the school nurse has changed dramatically in the last ten years as changes in society have taken place. As a result, there is an increased demand for health services in schools. The days of just applying bandages and assigning nurses to cover multiple schools are in the past.

Today's professional school nurse has a diverse and challenging role. Under the requirements of federal law, more disabled students than ever before attend public schools.

Procedures such as tracheotomy suctioning, bladder cauterization, ostomy care, gastric feedings, and ventilator care are now all part of the school nurse's daily responsibilities. School nurses are uniquely qualified to handle the care of students with specialized medical needs, in addition to the children with chronic conditions, such as asthma, diabetes, and life-threatening food allergies.

School nurses working in the public schools are required to be registered nurses, preferably with a bachelor's degree in nursing or working toward a degree, and have three years of experience in pediatrics. They receive licensure from the Department of Education and are required to pass the communication and literacy skills test. The department has recently changed the requirements for professional licensure to include a master's degree or passing the National Examination for School Nurses.

Screenings for vision, hearing, oral health, scoliosis, height, weight, and body mass are done every year as a preventative measure to discover potential health problems. Injury and illness assessments are an integral part of each day. Schoolchildren often come to school with colds, strep throat, respiratory infections, sprains, rashes, and other complaints.

Nurses take vital signs, listen to lung sounds, assess pain, evaluate, examine, and execute interventions. Many parents rely on the school nurse's assessment to determine if their child should stay in school, return home, or see their pediatrician. For some families, the nurse is their only access to health care.

Injuries such as bumps, bruises, cuts, abrasions, pencil stabs, stapled fingers, poked eyes, bloody noses, finger jams, rolled ankles, and sprains are common. The presence of a school nurse accounts for 90 percent of students returning to class to resume their studies. When serious injury does happen, it can make all the difference to the medical outcome when a nurse is available to respond quickly.

Students with mental health issues are frequent visitors to the nurse, often to take medications or to seek out a safe place to relax when the rigors of schoolwork and social interactions become overwhelming. We are often first to identify mental health issues and start the referral process, where we collaborate with parents, teachers, guidance counselors, administrators, and clinicians.

As the health care expert within the school system, the school nurse plays a leadership role in coordinated school health programs. Nurses participate as members of health advisory councils and crisis-disaster management teams, both in and outside the school community. School nurses lend their voices to advocate for policy in local and state government on behalf of students and their families.

There are many more roles that school nurses fill that can be expanded upon. School nurses truly make a profound difference in their school communities and need your support whenever schoolchildren need our advocacy.

Linda Betley, MSN, RN
Massachusetts

The Many Hats of This Nurse

My rotation as a student nurse at the original Children's Hospital of Philadelphia forever guided my choice to be involved in some area of pediatrics as a lifelong career.

I landed in pediatric critical care in the middle seventies at a time when children were being discharged with technology that had never before been used in the home setting. Thus, children were no longer tethered to the hospital. Surgeries, medicine, diagnostic tools, and equipment meant that more children were surviving but were going home with more complex needs.

I work in a school district with over seventeen thousand students. The majority of our students receive free or reduced lunches. On a daily basis, we help our families with the many challenges of language, culture, frequent moves, extended family caretakers, transitioning or lack of health care, and a myriad of educational, health, and social issues.

We are active in our district with health promotion and wellness. The nurses are part of a district-wide wellness committee based on the components of a coordinated school health model. Each nurse participates on the wellness committee in her building. There are before- and after-school wellness activities for students and their families. There are health fairs, a weight loss incentive program, and flu shots for faculty. We just partnered with the Department of Health with the goal of giving free flu shots in school for students.

As one highly regarded author in the ranks of the National Association of School Nurses (NASN) put it, "What should come across loud and clear is that school nurses do it all." I speak for all school nurses when I say our work is not easy, but daily we have the opportunity for those healthy, teachable moments. Much time can pass before positive outcomes can be seen. We are involved in the student's education, family, physical, and mental health and treatment, and the school community. We can be involved in communications with school leaders—for example, the superintendent and the school board—and with all other staff who interact with students.

It is vital for the school nurse to communicate with the health care community and other social agencies that support our students and their families with their life challenges. Changes in state and federal laws that affect the education and the health of our students challenge us to maintain active membership in our local, state, and national school nurse organizations, attend conferences, and communicate with legislators, parents, and the media. For many years, our state has been trying to change the certified school nurse ratio of 1:1,500 students to that of 1:750 students, as recommended by NASN position statements and the nation's health objectives in Healthy People 2010. I join my fellow NASN colleagues in saying wholeheartedly, "Every child in every school deserves a school nurse." In my district, certified school nurses conduct health services of growth, hearing, vision, scoliosis, and review of immunizations and mandated exams. Daily visits to the health room for illness, injuries, and an ever-increasing number of psychiatric medications are complicated by chronic disease management and severe health issues. There are asthma, diabetes, and severe allergic reactions requiring the nurse to perform specialized procedures. All these chronic and severe health concerns require individualized health care plans. Children with chronic and complex health conditions and who are medically fragile require case management services. The school nurse partners with the services and staff in the community where these children receive care.

The nurses throughout our state are very active in safety at school. They are concerned with issues of the school environment, drugs and alcohol, mental health, disaster preparedness, and flu prevention. Many nurses volunteer on their local hospital committee for pandemic flu preparedness. Finally, our state requires that all school nurses obtain a certain number of "Act 48" credits for our Department of Education in order to maintain our certification as school nurses. Our state also recently passed a law that all nurses must obtain continuing education hours. We partner collegially with many professionals in order to keep abreast of the changes in the field of school nursing.

In summary, this is exactly what the school nurses of this state, who wear many hats, do day in and day out, year in and year out. Hats off to all my fellow certified school nurses!

Barbara L. Filer, BSN, RN, CSN
Pennsylvania

LITTLE DID I KNOW

I took this position as school nurse under the advisement of one of my good friends, who was also a school nurse. She said, "Look at it this way. You'd get every weekend off, every holiday off, your summers off with pay. It would be good for you." I would be taking over for her while she moved to a different school within our district. Little did I know everything that was in store for me at this particular school!

Here is a typical day for me. Arrival at school is at 7:30 a.m., and right off the bat I have eleven meds to hand out between 7:30 and 8:00 a.m. I am giving everything from Ritalin to K-Phos® to Focalin XR®. Then, teachers of the children come into my office to argue with me as to whether or not I gave the morning medication, because the child is "not acting right." I then have to explain that medication usually can take anywhere from thirty to forty-five minutes to start to take effect. After conversing with teachers, and if I don't have to chase down any kids to come and take their meds, I have tube feedings on two children in self-contained classes. They also have diaper changes. An aide does come to assist, but I have to be present. I also have one ten o'clock medication to administer.

Lunch rush happens next. From 10:45 a.m. to 12:05 p.m., I have to give eleven more medications; and at 11:30 a.m., I have a breathing treatment of Albuterol to administer. Then, I finally get lunch if I can get out the door without someone seeing me and calling me back. From 2:00 to 2:30 p.m., I have four afternoon meds to give. One little girl will not take her potassium without juice in it, so I have to make sure we keep a supply of juice handy for this purpose. This is all scheduled. I don't want to even talk about the number of pain relief network meds that I have to give.

There are over seven hundred children enrolled at my school and only one of me. We have four other RNs and one LPN within our district. Everyone tries to cover for each other when someone is sick or out with a personal issue, but my school requires that a nurse be present at all times due to the fact that we have two very serious diabetics. One requires Accu-Cheks® at ten o'clock, noon, and two o'clock. His glucose levels are frequently off; they are either too low or too high, and then I have to call his mom about the situation because he needs to go home. The other student's check is at noon. He is usually very on the mark with his levels. Mom does well by him.

The other reason for a constant nurse is our two tube-feeding, wheelchair-bound students. They get fed at nine thirty and ten o'clock, and then again at one thirty and two o'clock. Usually one is after the other. We also have six other children with autism, as well as other learning disabilities. Someone is always getting bitten or scratched. There are numerous asthma patients that come in frequently to use their asthma pumps, which are left in a cabinet for them. I'm up to twenty-two asthma pumps.

On a typical day, I see anywhere between seventy-five and one hundred twenty children in my office for any given reason, and this does not include the meds and feedings. Kids come out of the woodwork. They scratch on bug bites till they bleed. They pull off scabs to come and get Band-Aids. They wet themselves, and it is up to me to either find clothes or call the parents—and that's not always kindergarteners. Fourth graders also do this act just to get to go home. You can always tell when there is a substitute in the classroom because you see the whole class for some reason or the other. They put stuff into their ears and up their noses. They want me to be a twenty-four-hour pharmacy. I can't give out any medications other than the prescribed ones— no Tylenol or Pepto. Everyone knows this, but they still come.

I have heard it has always been like this. I thought it was because I was new. That burst my bubble. I love working with kids, though, and I thought this would be great experience and a good opportunity for me.

Tracy Jones, RN
Arkansas

KNOCK-KNOCK

It is still early days for me as a practicing school nurse; however, I continuously find it very rewarding, despite the challenges that it can and does bring. As the sole school nurse for pre-kindergarten through second grade, many complaints, stomachaches, or "Oops! I wet my pants" events come through the door to our health room. Sometimes all it takes is a quick call to talk with mommy to hear her voice, which magically relieves the phantom stomachache. Then there is the quick fix to wash off the blood, apply a bandage, and wipe the tears after a fall on the playground. Thank goodness we have enough Band-Aids on hand to save the day, even if my old eyes cannot see the cut when the child swears, "It's right there!" Sometimes it takes an exchange of knock-knock or chicken jokes to relieve the anxiety or tension felt from an accident, a classroom exercise, or substitute teacher syndrome.

Being a school nurse has brought me to a venue that constantly reminds me of a gentleman from my formative years: Art Linkletter. I recall this entertainer having a segment on his television show where "kids say the darnedest things." Being a school nurse, you quickly learn that kids do say the darnedest things or provide more information than we need to know.

Our school has a program in which our children eagerly participate. Children learn to compose letters, address envelopes, and deliver the mail within the school itself. It has been pure delight to be on the receiving end of this mail system. The letters I have received are gracious, amusing, and provide a feeling of self-worth for one's nursing efforts. For instance, one student writes how she wished I was with her on vacation when she lost a couple of teeth. She reports that they did not have the little envelopes to place her lost teeth in. "My mom put them in her change purse with her dimes and pennies until we returned home." Then there are the letters that compliment your magic nursing skills. For instance, one student wrote, "You always know how to make my boo-boos go away." Another student reported, "I think my cut went down the drain with the soapy bubbles and water in your office. I can't find it anywhere."

Then there are the discussions about Santa, the Tooth Fairy, the Easter Bunny, and so on. This is where the children bring the magic to me. I am entertained by the enthusiasm these fantasy figures give them. Imagination only lasts a few years, and the children outgrow it way too soon. It makes your heart leap with joy to hear them discuss their own family traditions and the kindness shown to each other. I have learned over the years many different ways to cook, stuff, and carve a turkey. I did not realize how much a turkey enjoys a bubble bath before you fry it in the microwave for two hours.

The challenges begin on the first day of school and can linger for weeks at a time. These include being away from a parent for hours and riding a bus to a building other than home with a bunch of children that you never met before. And hey, who's that driving this big yellow thing anyway? Let the stomachaches begin!

School nursing is no joke; I take my job very seriously. However, timing is everything, isn't it? That's especially true when you have taken care of twenty-five-plus students and it's only eleven o'clock. By this time in a typical day, some of the treatments involved a serious head injury, possible arm fracture, multiple requests for use of inhalers because "we're going to gym right now," and a vomiting episode that missed the wastebasket and scored on your shoes. It is then when a good knock-knock or chicken joke would do a world of good. By the way, did you hear the one about …?

Patricia A. DeLorenze, LPN
Connecticut

School Nursing in a Rural Community

I work as a school nurse in a rural school of eighty-three students, grades kindergarten through twelve. Our school doesn't have the funding to staff a full-time registered nurse. Rather, I am employed hourly to accomplish the tasks required by the state.

Rural communities especially can benefit from a full-time school nurse. Schools are the center of all small-town activities, and sometimes are the only resource families have. Low-income families are part of what make up rural communities, and many families don't have health insurance. These communities are often underserved and can be quite a distance from any means of health care. For some families, this means going without. The school nurse is sometimes the only health care professional a family has. She can do a lot of assessment and refer children to their physician as needed.

There are many resources available for children who are in need of health care and cannot afford it. In the school I worked in during college, the full-time RN was able to bring resources to her community. One example is the Ronald McDonald bus that she brought from a nearby city. Families were able to come to the school that day and have dental care done, whether they had insurance or could afford it or not.

Working on an "as needed" basis and not having funding for school nursing projects is a struggle I deal with as a rural school nurse. As a nurse, my instinct is to do as much as possible to help the children and community, whether it is finding resources for them to get the care they need or providing education on health topics.

One advantage of working with only eighty-three students is that one can get to know the students well, and when a big issue does arise, it doesn't go unnoticed. But with me not being there on a regular basis and working with a faculty that does not understand the role of the school nurse, it may be quite some time before I get a call asking for my help. This was the case when a high school boy participating in sports and physical education had untreated ringworm for two weeks before I was notified. This also happened with a high school girl who had methicillin-resistant staphylococcus aureus (MRSA) all over her body. She had been seen by a doctor—without a follow-up—and continued to participate in physical education even after the MRSA had spread to her face and hands. Fortunately, in both cases, no other students were infected before these students obtained appropriate care. I learned after these instances that I needed to educate the faculty on my role and availability.

While there are struggles working as a school nurse in a rural area, it can also be very rewarding. The most rewarding is being that trusted adult that the students can come to about anything. It does help that I am still in my twenties and, for some time, actually went to school with some of the students. Whether it is with a pregnant girl or the student who was transferred to our school leaving all of her friends behind, it feels good to know that I helped, even if it was only a small amount, by just listening and being there for them. I just wish that I could be there for the students on a regular basis, even if it was just one or two mornings per week. Although it is sometimes difficult working as a school nurse in a rural area, it is so rewarding to help in any way that I can. Helping others is definitely worth overcoming any obstacles.

Anne E. Allen, BSN, RN, OCN
Montana

Baseline Data

School nursing is far from "boring," as some people believe. Day in and day out, year after year, loving what you do for those you care for averts boredom or monotony. Anyone who understands "same but different" understands that each child comes with their own uniqueness. The necessity of maintaining a healthy and safe school environment requires the school nurse to perform daily routine services, as well as handling all emergencies. In viewing baseline data stories, one will find it hard to imagine anyone being able to accomplish all that is required of one person in a single day. Yet this is exactly what school nurses do, day in and day out, year after year.

WAITING TO BE BORED

We are one of the few states that mandate school nursing. Unfortunately, it is an underfunded mandate. This means that school districts must have certified school nurses with a ratio of no more than one nurse to every fifteen hundred students. Districts are reimbursed for these services and medical and dental services, but the average district only sees reimbursement for about 23 percent of the cost of these services. Our school code was enacted in 1949. I wasn't born yet. Over the years, things have been added, but the ratio remains the same.

So, here I am today doing a job I love. My husband lovingly calls me "mother to the world" or at least to the 3,100 school kids I provide school health services to and to the twenty thousand kids I support as district department chair for health services. My state mandates that a school nurse must be an RN with a BSN and must complete a certification program of school nursing at one of twenty universities or colleges. When I left the neo-natal intensive care (NICU) facility, the neonatologist said, "You will be bored." I am still waiting and hoping for boredom to set in. A nice boring day would be good about now. Yes, I went to college for this.

Today they brought Susan to me. She was scratching her arm, making "z" cuts and cross patterns in the tender skin just above her inner wrist, scratches deep enough to bleed. She sees nothing wrong with this behavior.

I remember her as a little girl when I was her elementary school nurse. At that time, Susan informed me that she was not even tall enough to reach the clothesline, so she jumped with each piece of clothing to grab the line and hang on while she pinned the clothes.

Today, she says she does all the housework. Things haven't changed although they did move to a new house. Guidance is involved, and the county was called. I washed her arm gently and put Band-Aids on her wrists, hugged her, and asked her to please let us help. Off she went, and I was left with a deep sense of exhaustion.

Too bad I had no time to recoup. Other kids are waiting, and they want someone interested in them and focused on their needs. So I take a deep breath, then I calm, pat, smile, and listen.

Another student doesn't like art, just wants to rest, and comes to do just that. I give them twenty minutes, and then it's back to class.

An emergency! A student had a seizure on the bus while on the way to school and is now in the ambulance on the way to the hospital.

Teachers stop by for blood pressure checks and advice, and the day goes on.

A bat is loose in the hall. The custodian is chasing it, and the kids are screaming. The custodian asks for hair spray to slow down the bat. Hair spray!

In between kids, I check bid sheets and call nurses to verify their requests and write up purchase orders for special supplies. I call to check on CPR recertification and other problems and schedule my trip out of town tomorrow to learn about support services for my pregnant and parenting teens. More kids come into my office for medical van appointments, Band-Aids, rest, and pills. Parents, too, come looking for help and support. I am the best PR this school ever had, but no one knows it but me. Finally, it's time to go home.

The next day, I am at a conference. I learn how to use the computer program to record the statistics. The result of all this will be grant money to provide transportation to school for the moms and their babies. No, I am not making it easier for kids to have babies. I am making it easier for them to stay in school and graduate. I get out early and stop by school to get my mail. First mistake!

The possibly pregnant girl listens to me. She is on Ritalin but spoke to Planned Parenthood and is holding her medications until she sees the doctor. Now she is ready to have me talk to her mom.

Tomorrow the van comes, and with any luck the other pregnant girl—who emphatically states she is a "virgin"—will come to school and see the doctor. Friends report they have felt the baby move.

The pregnant girl never showed up for the van appointment, so it is time for guidance and the administration to get involved. The young man with the seizure is still in the hospital. Today is quiet; we only have a half day. I am making a list of all the extra things I do, and so far I have thirty things on the list. I spend the afternoon cleaning up and organizing the office.

New day, new problems ...

I manage to get a student a dentist appointment. It took three calls to reach the insurance company, yet we managed to get an appointment on Monday, less than one week from now.

Health services will provide first aid and blood pressure checks for the community.

Now, I have a meeting with community agencies about the resource room. This is a new initiative to provide on-campus mental health support groups. Let's hope I can pull this off.

The student is out of the hospital and came to school to get the medication straightened out. I am the basic health gatekeeper.

Nice weekend, but you would never know I was off. We hit the ground running, stomachaches and headaches. The pregnant girl is not pregnant; the teachers are dumbfounded. Another abuse report, and the family services agency is called. They are busy but will come after lunch.

A kid shows up to get ice for his friend in gym class. Okay, here is the ice, but I need to see the kid. The friend shows up again. Do you have crutches? No, I do not, so I run to the gym with a wheelchair, call the mom, and do the paperwork; then I orient the student nurse, who is having her community health experience with big eyes and her mouth hanging open.

Time for the IEP (individual education plan) meeting: the principal volunteers to stay in the health room while I run to the IEP meeting. I run, and the meeting ends because the kid decides to get his equivalency diploma. The principal tosses me the keys and says, "Never again. I can't do this." He runs away.

The gym student's ankle is in a cast. He broke it yesterday. Mom wants bussing, and I explain what we need for that to happen. Mom is happy because by two o'clock I have the bus arranged.

Another student doesn't feel good, and it is my fault. I leave messages with the parents; meanwhile, the student goes to art to paint. Mom shows up, but the student is not in class, and now the stories start. There was a strange boy here looking for her. There was a car accident. Everyone is running around, while she is at home sleeping. She decided she needed to rest and just left.

Meanwhile, someone else wants a hug, a boy hides his medicine, and I have to check his mouth and call Dad.

This is a big day, with sixty-nine students in school physicals. The school doctor is nice and calm. A hockey stick to the mouth interrupts the school physicals. The dentist's appointment I arranged was forgotten. A girl needs some of her Ritalin. She "lost" her pill in the park, and I start looking for Mom.

Then the afternoon fun begins. I get the student a new appointment with the dentist. The insurance lady says, "It is nice of you to help the student." Yes it is, but this is my job. Clean up the fight injuries, and do the paperwork on the physicals.

Tomorrow is another day.

This all happened. I used to keep a journal, because I know no one would believe all this. My husband thought it was funny. I was too tired to keep writing. I chose sleep. I love this despite all the heartaches, because I know that every day, I make the difference in the life of at least one student.

Kathleen M. Halkins, BSN, RN
Pennsylvania

3,659 and Counting

What *does* that school nurse do all day? I had my own perception before I engaged in this role three years ago, and I can tell you that I didn't even come close to reality. This is a job that you can't quantify, but I would like to attempt to define this role with some facts, figures, and thoughts.

From September 6, 2007, to May 31, 2008, the following statistics hold true:

- Students have lost close to one hundred teeth. Ninety-eight to be exact. One student lost three teeth in one day. That's a record! By the way, the going rate per tooth as per the Tooth Fairy is five dollars.
- I took approximately eight hundred temperatures.
- The number of adhesive dressings (also known as "Band-Aids") applied was approximately seven hundred.
- Every student has been screened for height, weight, and blood pressure. The biggest growth spurt was five and three-quarters inches in one year by a fifth grader. That's a new record!
- Fourth-grade students have had vision screenings as per state requirements.
- Third-grade students have had hearing screenings as per state requirements.
- Student visits to my office total 3,659. That averages out to approximately twenty-two students per day. Add on the ten visits by my daily students with medical needs, and you can see that getting through a day is quite a task. The most children seen in one day were fifty-two.
- Third and fourth graders have had six health lessons each. Fourth-grade girls have had a menstruation lesson. Fifth-grade boys and girls have had a puberty lesson.

I wear *many* hats. Among them are psychiatrist, surrogate mother, seamstress, housekeeper, wardrobe malfunction engineer, attitude adjuster, horticultural therapist, shoulder to lean on, "Can you fix this?" resource (eyeglasses, shoes, etc.), infection controller, splinter remover, hygiene supervisor, dentist, and many more. I have dried their tears, held their hands, provided comfort to their wounds (physical and otherwise), and laughed with them about their antics. They tell the best stories!

I am so fortunate to be part of the outstanding school team. My colleagues are awesome.

By the time my lunch rolls around at one o'clock, I am long overdue for a respite. And I do the best for myself to recharge. Ready or not, I return to my office to finish out the day. You wouldn't believe how many students visit me in the last thirty-five minutes. It makes me wonder how they survive without me!

There are days when I just go home and collapse, that is, as long as my family allows. There are days when I just can't get a situation out of my head. And it seems that my mind comes up with brilliant ideas at 4:00 a.m.! There are days when my sadness runs deep. There are days when I walk on cloud nine, knowing that I have made a difference in the life of a child. That's when I know that I am where I am meant to be.

And I didn't even scratch the surface of keeping up with an ever-changing world when it comes to health issues that impact my school nurse practice. I spend hours of time involved in committee work within my school and within the district. This keeps me busy in pursuit of optimal performance.

I know I have overlooked many things, but for now, I believe this is a great start to understanding the vital role that a school nurse plays every day.

In closing, I would like to remind you that I work with eleven other women who are responsible for our six thousand district students. Would you like to know what they do?

Carol Ann Scalgione, RN
New Jersey

No Monotony Here

A parent once asked me, "How can you stand to deal with all of those whining adolescents with the same complaints, day after day, year after year? Isn't it monotonous? Aren't you bored?" My first feelings were defensive and angry, but as I thought about it, I realized how little that parent knew about what I actually do and experience in my profession as a school nurse in a middle school. In fact, I do see students in the same age groups, day after day, year after year, but that is where the "sameness" ends.

As with our own children, students are wonderfully different people, with individual thoughts, feelings, and needs. They are filled with wonder and abilities to explore, struggle, and learn. In addition, they want to hurry up and grow up, while simultaneously they fear that they won't be children anymore. Their growth, day to day, is an ongoing adventure that I, as their school nurse, am fortunate enough to assist, nurture, and witness.

Teaching health classes is a part of my daily routine that allows me to experience and learn (in a different environment) about all of the students in my school. In addition, as the sole health care professional providing health services to seven hundred plus students, along with faculty and staff, I take care in meeting individual physical and emotional needs, while juggling the demands of mandated state and county paperwork requirements.

I am never "bored" as a school nurse, and I am fortunate to admit that my work is far from monotonous. My students are gifts, and they offer hope to us all that our future will be blessed with good things.

Jeanmarie Ringwood, MA, RN, CSN
New Jersey

From 7:00 a.m. to 3:30 p.m.

I am a school nurse responsible for the school health needs of four thousand students in eight school buildings. Today, I start at my high school at 7:00 a.m. Upon arrival, I make sure my cell phone is charged and the pager is on. When checking my e-mail, I find requests from two teachers at two of my elementary schools. One has a student who needs glasses but has no insurance; the other is regarding a student who has frequent absences due to asthma. My reply is, "We will address the issue on my next scheduled visit in two days' time" to the teacher who has the concern about vision. If the family does not have insurance to cover vision care and their income falls within the guidelines for a special vision care program, I can provide a gift certificate for a free eye exam and glasses for the student. I then write myself a note to call the teacher about the student with asthma when the elementary day starts at 8:30 a.m.

Meanwhile, two high school students are waiting at my door. One was in a car accident a few days ago and received stitches in his arm and scalp. The wounds are bandaged, but he requests a sling due to a sore shoulder. I question him as to whether the shoulder injury was apparent when he was in the emergency room, and he says that they did an X-ray that was normal. They gave him a sling and prescribed Motrin, but he left the sling at home today. I apply a sling to his arm, and he is ready to go to class.

The second student says she is feeling dizzy and her stomach hurts. She says she felt this way when she woke up, but it is final exam week and she has two exams today. I check her temperature, and it is 101.9 degrees. I call her home, but the only person home is her mother, who speaks only Arabic and does not drive. The student speaks to her mother and finds out that her older sister will be available to pick her up at nine o'clock. In the meantime, I make the student comfortable in the cot room until her family can arrive and notify her teachers that she is unable to take her exams today.

The morning continues with a steady stream of students who have a myriad of issues. Some come in with seemingly minor maladies that often turn out to be much more. I am very aware that during my three mornings at the high school, fewer students sign out to go home and are staying in school to learn. In addition, I frequently see staff members, who ask for blood pressure monitoring and health advice. In between seeing students and staff, I am doing paperwork to maintain health and immunization records. I also field questions about a few students' health histories in relation to special education eligibility and am invited to two upcoming student study team meetings.

At nine o'clock, I finally have time to call the elementary teacher about the student with asthma. She tells me that the student has missed thirty days of school to date and his mother says his asthma is the main reason. We decide to meet with the mother after school tomorrow. I am frustrated because if I had more time at each school, I could monitor absences more closely and intervene before it gets to the point of a possible truancy referral.

Around eleven o'clock, I get ready to leave the high school and go to one of my elementary schools. Just as I am about to go out the door, my pager goes off. It is one of the middle schools, and they have a student who has self-tattooed an image on her foot. They would like me to come and check it, and I agree to stop on my way to my afternoon school. Fortunately, there are no signs of infection, and the student tells me that she did this a week ago. The area is still a bit red, but healing well. I review the signs of infection with her, and we talk about how the skin is our barrier against infection; opening the skin greatly reduces its ability to protect us from infection. The counselor has already called her parent about the tattoo, but I call again to review signs of infection with her.

Back in my car, I am happy for a few minutes of quiet and a chance to eat my sandwich. While I am driving to my next school, my cell phone rings, and it is the assistant principal from the high school. He reports that a student took two pills from another student, who had them in a plastic bag. The student thinks they were Xanax, and he took them because he was feeling anxious. Returning to the high school, I do an assessment, and we try to locate the student who gave the pills to his friend.

It is now twelve thirty, and I am over an hour late to my elementary school. So much for best-laid plans: Some days I feel like I provide "drive-by" school nursing. After the pills are identified at the high school and I ensure that the student does not need emergency care and parents are on their way, I depart for the elementary school.

I arrive at the elementary school at 1:15 p.m. and realize that lunches are over in all my buildings and that I didn't get any calls regarding the ten diabetic students who take insulin at lunchtime. Anxiously, I hope that no news is good news and that the nonmedical staff members I trained have correctly monitored and provided care for the students.

Fortunately, things are pretty quiet at this elementary school today, so I spend my afternoon following up with parents of students who did not pass the hearing screening. We also have vision screening coming, so I notify teachers of this and ask for referrals from the grades not scheduled to be screened this year. This school has two classrooms for autistic students and two classrooms for students with emotional difficulties. I stop in those classrooms to see if there is anything new with any of the students. More checking and answering e-mail messages, and before I know it, it is 3:30 p.m. and time to go home. Tomorrow will be totally different because I will be in at least two or three other schools. One thing is for sure: this job is never boring!

Laurie Feldkamp, BSN, RN
Michigan

Back and Forth Between Schools

Prior to entering the field of school nursing, I really had no idea what a school nurse did. I wasn't sure if it was the right career choice for me. I started by working as a substitute for the last few weeks of a school year. I was then hired to work permanently the next year. When I began, two district nurses covered seven school buildings. I have now worked as a school nurse for twelve years, ten as a certified school nurse. Currently, I cover a middle school and an elementary building. My two buildings are located in the same block, and combined I have approximately eleven hundred students.

While my caseload has decreased, the biggest challenge of my job continues to be managing children's healthcare when I must split my time between two buildings. Health conditions like asthma, food allergies, seizures, ADHD, diabetes, and bleeding disorders are the most common issues that must be monitored and treated within my school setting. It is vital that school staff be trained to monitor these conditions and identify symptoms that require attention. Many times the medical condition can require immediate action, such as the administration of medication. Unfortunately, this responsibility may fall to the principal or other school staff when the nurse is not in the building. Training and a thorough care plan can assist these nonmedical personnel in carrying out these responsibilities.

During the past school year, I had three diabetic students in one building and one in another. Combined, they had three different lunchtimes. While I made every attempt to get where I needed to be, there were times when another situation would require my attention. In these cases, I relied on secretaries and principals to ensure that students were checked and that their blood glucose levels were measured. Insulin dosages at times were calculated and communicated over the phone. However, some students that required an injection had to wait for me to arrive, resulting in delay in insulin action, missed class time, and the frustrated feeling of not being able to do everything that everyone needs at the same time.

Because you get to know your students so well and know their conditions, you are like a worried parent when you are not at school to take care of them. While we have a few substitute nurses that can be called when we are unable to work, there are often times when they are not available. In that case, one of the other two nurses in the district must cover the responsibilities of the absent nurse, with assistance from the principals and secretaries. I often call the secretaries at my schools on sick days or conference days to check on students and make sure medications have been administered.

While the busy days of walking back and forth between schools in the rain and snow can often be frustrating, I am fortunate to work with a caring and responsible staff that is willing to make sure each student's health is a priority. As a school nurse, you have the ability to comfort, assist, treat, advocate, and educate. Sometimes you get to see the results of your efforts, and sometimes you don't. When you do, it can be incredibly rewarding. You get to know a lot about students and their families and develop lasting friendships. I love my job, and I look forward to the challenges of school nursing that lie ahead.

Sherri Verdun, BS, RN, CSN
Illinois

Big Luxuries in a Little Town

Being the school nurse in a small, rural community gives me the opportunity and the luxury to spend quality time with students. I serve approximately three hundred students, ranging in age from preschool through twelfth grade. Having such a wide range of ages keeps me busy with multiple teaching opportunities along with the everyday boo-boos and piles of paperwork.

The beginning of every year is busy with making sure all students are current with their immunizations. I write many notes to remind families of immunization deadlines each and every year. Thanks to the state immunization registry, I am able to access immunization records over the Internet to help me with this feat. At the end of every year, I also send home letters to parents of sixth graders and all incoming kindergarteners to remind families of what immunizations are needed for their child to attend school. Taking an active role in "kindergarten roundup" helps me to become acquainted with the incoming kindergarten parents. This helps to make the beginning of the year a little more organized, and it is hoped that those students received their required immunizations over summer break.

At the start of every year, I also make sure that the health information form is filled out on every student. I then have knowledge of allergies, health concerns, emergency contacts, and such. Multiple parent contacts are made at the beginning of every year to clarify any information on the forms. Even though we are a small school, student health can change over summer break, so a new form must be filled out every year.

During every year, I teach multiple topics, including hand washing, to promote child health to preschool through second grade. This yearly reinforcement helps the students to remember how to wash their hands. I also do some health teaching along with this; I talk about how to help prevent the spreading of germs, which cause sickness. I present a unit of information called "Medicines in My Home" to sixth graders. At this age, these students start to self-medicate. This presentation stresses the importance of reading medicine labels and making sure to include parents and guardians in any decision concerning medicines. It is hoped that this will help decrease the number of students who abuse medications, while the unit also teaches about the safe use of medications. In the spring of every year, I also do the "puberty talk" with the fifth grade girls and arrange for a male speaker to come speak with all of the fifth-grade boys on this subject.

Every year is busy with performing health screens on many of the students at my school, as well as with helping the other five schools in our district.

Another important job is to inform the cooks of any food allergies, making sure that families have obtained notes from the doctor that specify food substitutions if necessary and that these notes are on file. Additionally, I have to make sure that those asthma students who carry an inhaler with them have the appropriate permission sheet filled out and on file.

In addition to school health screenings, I perform initial drug evaluations on suspected students and call in the school resource officer if needed. Head lice screening is done on an as-needed basis. Suspected students are checked. If they are positive, their siblings are checked, as well as others in their class. And, being in such a small school, I could end up checking the entire school! Throat swabs for strep throat are also done, with parental permission as needed.

Being a liaison for parents/guardians, doctors, therapists, and students, along with being an advocate for the students and the parents, are other important responsibilities that I have. Other responsibilities include: attending multiple meetings throughout the year, such as IEP, 504, or BIT meetings, gathering information from teachers of students with attention deficit hyperactivity disorder to forward to their doctor for medication review appointments, making abuse/neglect referrals to the Department of Family Services, making referrals for those students who fail the school screenings, and compiling and sending home letters to all parents about current health issues or outbreaks as the need arises.

Not only do I dispense medications, but I have the luxury to give a lot of TLC. I change clothes when a young kindergartener has had an accident or when a student has fallen in a water puddle at recess. I fix glasses for the students whose lenses have fallen out and mend zippers (sometimes using a paper clip as the zipper pull). I remove chewing gum from hair, and sometimes even brush and wash hair. I style young girls' hair for those who need a little pick-me-up, apply Band-Aids to those imaginary boo boos, and clip the first-grade guinea pig's nails when needed.

Working in a small school allows me to also help out in many other non-nursing ways. These include after-school bus duty, recess duty, and inside lunch duty. I answer the phone, take attendance, and watch the classes when the teachers need some extra help. I am also in charge of checking the temperature and weather for the elementary students who hope to go outside for recess. Along with this, I hand out borrowed coats, hats, and mittens for those who need them for recess. We also have students with health concerns, including asthma and diabetes.

One thing I truly enjoy is being able to make a student smile. I had a first-grade student who came to school with gum in her hair. I got vegetable oil from the cooks to get the gum out, washed her hair, and nicely combed it.

Her face shone for the rest of the day. Many compliments were given by the staff, which made her feel even better.

The "Ten Commandments of School Nursing" by an unknown author sums it up:

1. You get more headaches when the weather is nasty. Everything hurts more when it's raining.
2. A substitute teacher is good for at least three stomachaches.
3. *Everything* is contagious in first grade, even sprained ankles.
4. The shrine at Lourdes will never be responsible for as many miracles as the three o'clock bell.
5. Practically every serious school-time injury occurs when Mother is at the store.
6. Paper cuts are more painful to children under seven years of age. Even the invisible cuts need a Band-Aid.
7. Children think they are supposed to throw up in the water fountain.
8. Never keep good-tasting cough drops in your office.
9. A school nurse should never expect to eat a hot lunch.
10. Because children think they should always have access to you, *never, ever,* go into the bathroom without locking the door.

But, having the luxury to spend quality TLC time with the students is irreplaceable.

Candi Thomas, BSN, RN
Wyoming

A Day in the Life of a School Nurse

I work at a large high school with 1,675 students and one hundred faculty and staff. I also service the alternative school next door (fifty students) and the central office. My day begins at 7:45 a.m. Some days I have students follow me in the building to take care of an injury that happened last night. Mom wants to know if it is broken or if they need stitches. I administer early morning medications for a few students that will not remember to take them at home.

I return phone calls left on my answering machine from parents. Then I start getting busy! In a day, I will see an average of forty-five students who have acute and chronic illnesses and injuries. I have a rule about sending students home. To qualify for going home, their temperature must be over one hundred degrees, or they must have vomiting or bleeding I cannot stop. I really am not quite that strict, but I like the students to think I am.

On "club days," I have a diabetes support group of twenty students that meet. I also have a teen pregnancy and parenting support group that meets once a month.

We have a drug-testing program that is implemented by the school nurses. I try to drug test six to ten students every day. On some days I may do as many as twenty five, as I need to do approximately three hundred fifty students three times a year. I also test the faculty and staff from a random testing pool.

Sometimes I spend most of the day doing health education in the ninth-grade health class. I educate four hundred twenty students about: sex education, anatomy of reproduction, sexually transmitted diseases and AIDS, healthy hearts, and healthy lifestyle choices.

During the day, I will get several e-mails from nurses across the state that have health issues and concerns. I have held many positions on the state board for several years.

During flu season, I give several students and faculty flu shots. I am one of the CPR and first-aid instructors for the school district. I certify about eighty staff every year. I send out all the immunization letters for updates, and I record all the information in the computer.

The nurses in my district do all the special needs training. I see many mental and social problems with students daily. These kinds of problems cannot be fixed very easily, maybe not at all.

I do weight, height, and body fat index for the wrestling team. I do vision and hearing screenings for special education students and any other screening requests from teachers or parents. On a good day, things start slowing down around two thirty, and then I have time to finish up charting and having conference calls with parents and doctors.

I think most school nurses see very similar problems. I love my job, but it can be very overwhelming in the scope of things. May God bless all school nurses!

Phyllis Gentry, RN
Kentucky

The Hardest Job I Have Ever Loved

It is 7:00 a.m., and I am entering my "Thursday" school and getting myself mentally prepared for the day. As a school nurse with an assignment of four schools (two elementary, one middle, and one high school, with a combined population of over five thousand students), it does take some time to get "reprogrammed" for each new day. This is one of my elementary schools, and as I walk into the office, I see the normal morning hustle and bustle going on. I enter the clinic and pick up my folder, where my invaluable clinic assistant has placed my mail, updates regarding student concerns, the weekly report, and other miscellaneous papers. I hear taps on the window as students begin to stream by and wave on their way to class. The clinic door opens, and the day begins!

In rolls one of my most medically fragile students: a wheelchair-bound second grader with an infectious smile. It is great to see him so animated and full of excitement while telling me about a recent adventure. Other students begin to arrive with medication refills, notes from parents, and clinic passes. My assistant brings us both coffee, and we attempt to catch up on a week's worth of information as we tend to the children's needs.

Ahh ... the life of a school nurse; it is the life of kissing boo-boos and putting on Band-Aids ... *not*! I am always amazed when I talk to parents, teachers, and other individuals in the community about how little they understand the role of the school nurse. I describe it as one of the hardest positions I have ever loved. Today's school population includes an increasing number of children with significant health problems, some of them life threatening. The nurse must be someone who can function well as an independent practitioner. Interpersonal skills and the ability to be an effective communicator are a must since the nurse is working with children, parents, medical professionals, faculty, and school administrators. The nurse must also have exceptional assessment and problem-solving skills since we do not have the availability of sophisticated medical technology at our immediate disposal. Flexibility and organizational skills are critical. I also have learned to trust my gut feelings.

Who would have thought that as a school nurse I would make more emergency lifesaving interventions than I had in all my years as a hospital-based nurse? I have often said that one day I would write a book entitled *I Couldn't Make This Stuff Up If I Tried!* I could never have predicted that at the very beginning of one school year, I would be faced with an eighth grader who came into the clinic complaining of a stomachache; she recently had a baby, and none of this information was communicated to the clinic.

Not only are we there for the students, but one time an individual from the neighborhood came running into the school office with blood all over her arm from broken glass. I have no idea why she came to the school, but it just so happened that I was there. I held pressure on her wound with a sanitary pad—the most absorbent item I had at my disposal—until the paramedics arrived. Trust me, the list goes on and on. Not only are there the physical issues to address, but the emotional and psychosocial needs are incredible. I remember telling my husband that at times I feel like I am in the Peace Corps in my own community.

As I took a sip of coffee, the clinic phone rang. The person on the other end of the phone identified herself as an employee of the epidemiology department of the county health department. The individual went on to say that a student at the high school assigned to me had died in the early morning hours from bacterial meningitis. She asked that I go to the high school and find out which students may have been in close contact with the deceased student because they might require prophylactic antibiotic therapy. I felt my stomach twisting, but instinctively my mind started with the questions: "Had 'student X' been to the clinic the previous day, and if so, what were her complaints?" "Who were the student's teachers, and how many classmates may have had close contact and require treatment?" "What did I even remember about bacterial meningitis?" And of course, I thought about how tragic this was for the student's family.

I quickly got my things together and told my assistant that I was needed at my "Friday" school and to page me if anything came up. I threw my "office in a bag" (suitcase with wheels) into the trunk of my car and grabbed my resource books from the backseat to quickly refresh myself on the disease. Thank heaven for cell phones and the fact that I kept a phone list of all my schools in the car.

I called my "Friday" school and asked to speak to the principal. I shared with him the news from the county health department and that I needed to get the names of the close friends of "Student X." The principal indicated that he would e-mail only those teachers who taught the deceased student, and he would carefully word it so as not to cause any alarm. The names were to be sent to my e-mail address. I also asked the principal to advise the guidance counselors of the situation at hand and to please locate an office where I could meet quietly with individual students. I assured the principal that I was on my way to the school and that I would come to his office as soon as I arrived to further discuss our plan of action. I also contacted my clinic assistant in the high school to let her know that I was coming there and that I would update her when I arrived. I then phoned my supervisor to advise her of the situation and what steps were in place up to that point. She immediately assured me

49

that she was on her way to help with this enormous and emotionally charged task.

It was now 8:20 a.m. I arrived at the high school and quickly went to see the principal. His secretary provided me a copy of the e-mail that had been sent. The guidance counselors soon arrived. I summarized the information that I had gleaned from my medical resources and the health department. The biggest concern from the counselors was how the disease was spread. I reinforced that since the disease is transmitted through droplets from the secretions of an infected person, unless an individual had had a recent "saliva exchange" (kissing, sharing food, drinks, lipstick, cigarettes, etc.), the likelihood of transmission was very small. I then shared my immediate priorities, which included: identifying those students who may have had close contact with their deceased classmate, interviewing those individuals to determine their level of exposure, and informing the parents as to their children's "risk status" and treatment recommendations. This information then needed to be communicated to the epidemiology department so that they would know how many doses of medication would be required. The health department was also putting together informational letters about the disease, which would be sent home that afternoon with each student. They were also going to send an individual to assist with a faculty meeting scheduled for after school. In addition, arrangements needed to be made for the assistance of grief counselors as well as a central information center because once word got out, there would be a barrage of questions from students, parents, faculty, and the press.

It was now shortly after nine o'clock, and my supervisor arrived. She went to speak with the principal and the other administrators, and I headed to the clinic. When I shared the circumstances of this tragic situation with my assistant, she was devastated. She told me that "student X" had not been in the clinic at all that week. I shared that I would be giving her the names of certain students that I would need for her to call down to the office space that I was provided. I also told her that she would need to be prepared for a busy day. I checked my e-mail, and the teachers had sent me the names of seventeen students. I pulled their emergency cards so I would have phone numbers to contact parents, and I grabbed a few boxes of Kleenex. My supervisor and I then headed to our quiet space, where we discussed our strategy in meeting with each student. We agreed that we, of course, needed to be compassionate, but at the same time, we needed to get specific information quickly as to whether or not there was a "real risk" of a recent exposure to the disease. Once we assessed the information, we would then contact the student's parent to advise of the situation and provide the parent an opportunity to ask us questions. Since we had many students to meet with, once we obtained what we needed and provided information and comfort to the student, they would then be taken to a guidance counselor for additional emotional support. We took a deep breath and felt that we were ready to call the first student down.

Each session was difficult. We calmly explained that their friend had become very ill the previous evening and had passed away in the early morning hours of bacterial meningitis. We explained how the disease was transmitted and asked if they had shared any food, drinks, lipstick, cigarettes, and so forth with their friend within the last few days. As mentioned earlier, we needed to ascertain this information quickly before each student reacted emotionally. We then called each parent. Most parents came to the school to comfort their child and to get reassurance from us. Upon completion of our first round of interviews, it was determined that seven students would require medication.

During the time that we were meeting individually with the seventeen students, the principal made a general announcement to the school staff that a member of the student body had passed away that morning from bacterial meningitis. Students who had a concern as to whether or not they may have been exposed to the disease were instructed to report to the clinic. Students were also encouraged to see their guidance counselor if they required any kind of emotional support as a result of hearing this very sad news. Kids poured into the clinic and the front office in a range of emotional states. Again, my wonderful clinic assistant was able to provide some order to the chaos, and additional grief counselors were available to assist in the clinic.

The day was an emotional blur. Had it not been for the coordinated teamwork and support from the school and community resources, I am not sure how we would have made it. Informational notices about bacterial meningitis, as well as the required medication permission slips, were delivered to the school. The health department informed my clinic assistant that she was to collect the signed permission slips the following morning and then the medication could be administered. Parents were given the option of receiving the medication from their physician if they preferred.

The school day was over, and it was now time for the mandatory faculty meeting. Again, information about how the disease is spread was shared, and the staff was reassured that their risk of exposure was extremely low. Many, many questions from the staff and faculty were asked and answered by the experts from the health department.

What a day! All of us involved spent some time after the faculty meeting to debrief. We discussed what worked and what did not. Our major recommendation was that for future crises, it would be better to communicate to teachers via e-mail the circumstances and to allow each teacher to share the knowledge in a more personal way. Teachers would be notified via an announcement to check their e-mails. I offered to put together a protocol based on our recommendations should such a situation ever occur again. This protocol is now part of our school nurse manual.

As I reflect on the events of this day, I am overwhelmed. I am convinced that what I learned from all my nursing experience gave me the structure I needed to make it through. All my skills were put to the test: assessing, critical thinking, planning, decision making, communicating, implementing, and evaluating. As a school nurse, I have learned that there is no such thing as a typical day. It is the hardest job I have ever loved!

Amy Jayne Barnes, MA, BSN, RN
Florida

School Nursing Versus Fear
of Working Nights

I started subbing for local school nurses in 1990 as a result of my fear that I would be working nights at age sixty-five in my community hospital. I met my predecessor in a bathroom while taking advanced cardiac life support certification, and she was thrilled that I was available to work as a school nurse.

In September 1992, I was hired as the new school nurse-teacher. With any nursing job I had previously, there was at least a three-month orientation before you were "safe" to act on your own. There was no orientation here. Talk about being shot out of a cannon my first day! I got through it with help from other school nurses. I also continued to work per diem nights as an administrative coordinator at my community hospital. Staying active in my state's school nurse and teachers' organization and continuing to work at the hospital provides me the information and skills to survive the daily emergencies that come up.

As the sole nurse-teacher, I travel between two schools throughout the day via a wooded path. When I started in 1992, there were about six hundred twenty-five students, and kindergarten classes ran half the day. Ritalin was the number one lunchtime medication, and a few inhalers were administered. In 2008, the population is just under five hundred, with three full-day kindergarten classes. My medication cabinet primarily contains Epi-Pens® and inhalers for students in pre-K through fourth grade, along with insulin and glucagon, and seizure and cardiac medications. Students in grades five through eight carry their inhalers and Epi-Pens®. These students also have individualized health care and emergency care plans. I also had tracheotomy care and g-tube feeds for a couple of years before the student transferred this past September.

Before I started in this role, I wondered what a school nurse-teacher does all day. I got my answer: triaging minor and major emergencies, answering questions from staff looking for medical advice or blood pressure monitoring, monitoring blood sugars, dispensing medication, listening to a child having a sad day, attending evaluation team meetings, and all the health-mandated screenings. I remind the staff and parents I am not a doctor and cannot make medical diagnoses, only nursing diagnoses. I have a weekly spot on our e-mail newspaper reporting the "illness of the week" and health promotions. Parents call in to see what is going around and wondering whether they should seek medical follow-up.

The first few weeks of September are difficult for anyone in this role because the families arrive with none of the required health information and they cannot understand why I am upset. I remind them that it is for their child's health and well-being (and my sanity) that everybody has up-to-date information.

Today's threats for children are bullying and obesity. We use health education, policies, and assemblies to remind children to respect and accept one another and to promote healthy eating and physical activity as lifetime skills. State and federal regulations mandate policies for schools, but unless the family accepts the changes and the government puts money toward education, it will be a struggle for all communities.

Over the past sixteen years, I have made great friends with parents and students. As a native Newporter, I drive over the bridge twice a day! Together, our school physician and I teach the puberty lesson to grade five students. We make it a huge event for the students with hype and grab bags. Former students say, "You are still here?" when they enroll their children, and they tell me their children are better behaved than they were.

When the parents go to the community hospital, they ask the staff "Is Renie here?" Working in both worlds is beneficial for me when an emergency arises and I need to send someone off to the ER. I talk to the desk secretary whom I used to work nights with and give reports to one of the many ER nurses whom I know and trust, and off goes my patient in need to the ER with all the information to be cared for on arrival.

The challenges and the rewards of being a school nurse-teacher are varied, and every day is different. Knowing that when I am here I make a difference to students makes it all worthwhile.

Renie Sullivan, MEd, BSN, RN
Rhode Island

Do Vegetarians Eat Animal Crackers?

"I would like something in pink in a size six, please," stated a kindergarten student looking for a change of clothes because she accidentally wet her pants on the first day of school. That was the first of many amusing, memorable moments during my seven years as a school nurse.

A hungry first grader told me once that he did not think he should eat the animal cracker I gave him because he was a vegetarian. I laughed for days about that one.

I had worked in a hospital, in a doctor's office, and in an outpatient cardiac testing unit before embarking on my journey toward school nursing. Pediatric nursing was not my background.

On the day I received my school nurse certificate, I thought to myself, "Self, you did it! The hard part is over, so now this should be easy." I had already been hired by a school district, so I did not even need to find a job. Boy, was I ever wrong: this job is anything but easy.

The toughest job you will ever love is an advertising slogan for our military. It is also how I describe my feeling for school nursing.

About five years into my new career, a teacher who is a friend of mine and I were having a conversation about how hard it is to find a substitute school nurse. I wanted to be able to take a personal day without having to worry about who will take care of my three hundred thirty children. I worry about them; they are my kids. Our district of twenty-four schools has very few nurse substitutes, so taking a day off—which you are entitled to—is somewhat difficult. My friend told me she thought it would be easy to find someone to substitute for me because, "After all, how hard is it to put on Band-Aids all day?" It was at that moment that I realized some people do not know much about what real school nurses do.

Each and every day I walk into my office, I never know what awaits me. In my head, I have a general plan of what I would like to accomplish, but things never seem to go as planned.

I have those tasks that I must do routinely and those situations I must handle as they present themselves. Yes, I do need to administer first aid when needed, but that is just a small portion of my day-to-day activities. I need to fill out annual immunization reports, annual TB reports, and medical waste audits. I order needed supplies and try to figure out how to work online requisition forms and complete individual health care plans (IHP) for students in need. I do TB skin testing on all new employees and students and call parents to request the required paperwork for their child with asthma.

I must get in touch with the parents of a student with diabetes because her blood sugar levels are extremely inconsistent. I call social services for a child who has an imprint of a belt buckle on her arm and then track down medical files for new students. I check the vision of a student having trouble seeing the blackboard from the first row, teach families about the importance of completing their child's vaccination series to prevent a problem, and give a crying child a dollar so he can buy his mom a flower from the Mother's Day plant sale. I help a parent who does not speak English fill out a form so his child gets much-needed medical attention.

During the holidays, I identify families in need and provide them with donated food so they will be able to eat and enjoy their time together. I call a parent whose child has chips, soda, and a cupcake for lunch and let them know this is not an acceptable meal. I try to reassure a fourth grader from a culturally private family that she is not going to die because she has just gotten her period for the very first time. I take out the singing battery-operated birthday frog and let it dance for the child, as this may be their only birthday celebration, and meet with our safety committee to formulate a plan on how to handle an active shooter in our building. I meet with a teacher and the principal concerning a grave medical diagnosis on a student who has been in our building for five years. I cry with my principal with gut-wrenching grief and try to decide how we will ever be able to tell our students about the tragic death of one of our teachers and the death of a former student who just completed his first year in middle school.

I write a plan (IHP) for a student who broke her arm cheerleading the previous week. I answer questions from a colleague about a medical issue she may be having. I teach classes about hand washing, puberty, taking a bath, dental hygiene, good touch and bad touch, and how to properly urinate in a urinal. I conduct scoliosis screenings on the fifth graders and check blood pressures, heights, and weights on all classes; I screen all students for vision problems, assessing for color blindness and proper eye muscle balance. I try to read and understand new laws and state codes and mandates in order to provide my students with the best medical care possible while at school.

I could go on, but I think by now you can see that my job is diverse, emotional, rewarding, occasionally frustrating, and most of all, it is much more than boo-boos and Band-Aids. To me it is all about knowing that perhaps I will be able to make a difference to just one child. Hopefully I can reassure them, keep them safe, and let them know that there is really someone who cares about them.

One day, one of our teachers shared a story with me about the day her class was discussing heroes. Most of the class identified policemen and firemen as their heroes, but one student raised his hand and said, "Mrs. Robson is my hero!" After I finished crying, I realized I had achieved my goal. I had made a difference in the life of one child. That makes putting up with all the Band-Aid comments manageable. It also makes me raise the bar. It makes me want to be someone else's hero too.

Lori E. Robson, BSN, RN, CSN
New Jersey

Critical Care

Happiness, sadness, love, and anger all add up to loving the job of school nursing. In these chapters, you will discover that school nursing is far from the carefree job the general public perceives. School nurses become so involved with the children under their care that nurses can become emotionally drained; yet at the same time, providing medical care to critically ill children has rewards beyond description. You will become mesmerized by the challenges and requirements that a school nurse faces each day caring for critically ill children, and yet she manages to maintain love for the vocation.

It Mattered to This One

Each year the daunting task of health screenings begins with the first couple of weeks of school. This year was going to be different. Several nurses on staff decided to go from school to school as a team to screen vision, hearing, height, weight, teeth, and blood pressure, and check for scoliosis. We set up screening stations and determined student flow to minimize confusion. Everyone had pens, pencils, and sticky notes, and the health folders were ready to be handed to the students to carry from station to station. Classes were scheduled to come to the health office every forty minutes. We were all set to go.

Everything was going like clockwork until one fourth-grade student was taken out of the "flow" because a nurse wanted to recheck his blood pressure before he left the area. As we each finished with students at our assigned stations, we would try to pick up the slack at another station that was getting backed up. As things slowed down, several nurses found the student who had been taken out, noting that he was missing a blood pressure recording. Finally, the nurses realized that several nurses had each checked this student's blood pressure at least twice because they had found it elevated and each wanted to do a recheck. Since this student only spoke and understood Spanish, he did not or could not tell any of the nurses that he had already had his blood pressure checked several times. It became apparent that the boy's blood pressure was further elevated each time someone rechecked it.

Wow, our "well-oiled machine" had a cog missing! It was decided that the mother would be notified of our findings and encouraged to take her son to the doctor as soon as possible. When the mom came to the health office to pick up her son, she was strongly encouraged to take her son to the doctor or the emergency room before going home and was given a medical referral form, which indicated the problem that had been identified. We all felt confident that we had convinced the mom that we had serious concerns about her son's elevated blood pressure.

The next day, the screening process began again at the same site. Before we started, we called the school office to find out if the boy we had referred was at school on this day. To our surprise, we were told that he was indeed in class.

I asked the interpreter (another RN) to call Mom and once again urge her to come get her son and take him to the doctor immediately. Mom came to the health office for her son.

A few days later, we learned that the boy had been air evacuated to a larger hospital. We were told that he had an emergency surgical repair and was doing well. This problem had not been previously identified because he had recently moved into our area.

The bottom line on this is that if we identify and are able to remediate just one health problem through mass screening, the screening has been worth both our time and effort. We have since identified at least three more students with severely elevated blood pressures that required surgical repair, and they all had good post-op outcomes.

Shirley Rodriguez, BSN, RN, CSNP
Arizona

Here's the Deal

When I was little, I would take a paper table napkin and fold it corner to corner. My mom would take two bobby pins and pin the napkin to the top of my head. It sounds a little goofy unless you're a poor farm kid who had to use your imagination to take you to the land of make-believe.

Actually, I thought my nurse's hat was pretty cool. I spent many hours caring for my brothers and sisters, who were kind enough to pretend they were sick. Not to mention the animals that became my patients. So, I was a weird kid. What can I say? No matter how weird I seemed, I knew at a young age that I wanted to be in the medical field, either in the science of animals or the science of people.

Those days of make-believe are long gone, but the memories will be there until my mind remembers no more. Never would I have thought that nursing would have taken me down this wonderful path of learning that led to a road of medical adventures.

In 1987, I was fortunate enough to be hired by a neurosurgeon. During the interview, Dr. Johnson was talking about a Stryker frame and one of his patients. I really couldn't let on that I didn't even know what a Stryker frame looked like, let alone what it was used for. He hired me anyway. It wasn't long before I knew the importance of a Stryker frame. That was just a small percentage of all the things I learned. As with the neurosurgical job, I had no idea what lay in store for me when I became a school nurse.

Dr. Johnson taught me many things, but one of the foremost things in my mind was that all people are unique and a positive attitude can affect every part of our being. Whether it was the little girl with the malignant brain tumor or the singer who had herniated discs in his neck, he made me realize that you face the problem head-on, face your fears, and deal with it.

Sixteen years later, I am working as a school nurse. To be honest, I never knew much about school nurses until I had children of my own and they started school. I decided that school nursing was the job for me. I could work close to bankers' hours and have the rest of the time with my children, including three months off during the summer. This aspect of school nursing was very appealing to me. Little did I know, like the neurosurgical job, school nursing entailed much more than I had imagined.

The first year of my school nurse career was the first and only time I was subpoenaed to court to testify because of head lice. The case was settled out of court. I never thought I'd be pulling nits out of hair for hours at a time just so a student would not miss any more school. You can't take some things too seriously or they become overwhelming. So when you go to the grocery store and hear a child tell his mom, "There's the school nurse. She checked us for head lice today," you can only smile and enjoy the innocence of children.

Then there is the other side of school nursing. There's the sadness and worry you see in a child's eyes as they talk about their parents getting a divorce. You notice the student who comes to school with soiled clothes and tangled hair. You find the little boy who doesn't have a dad to look up to and a mother who is trying hard to make ends meet. This would be a pretty carefree job if their emotional and psychological problems were as easy to remedy and as simple as putting on a Band-Aid. A school nurse cannot fix everything, but we sure do our best to try.

One of my favorite students encompasses every aspect of my job. "Jesse" comes from a single-parent family. His mom definitely loves him, which is evident by his loving and happy demeanor.

He was diagnosed with Type I diabetes at age five. The school system was not aware that he even existed, and so he did not start kindergarten until he was past age six.

Diabetes is challenging in and of itself, but when dysfunction is added into the equation, it can be even more so. Jesse sometimes comes to school with a blood sugar level over four hundred and is usually honest enough to tell you that he had a piece of cake or some corn chips before school. Perhaps if he had received insulin to cover what he ate that morning, his blood sugar would not be that high.

When Jesse started kindergarten, he stayed longer than the other students in order for the school to provide him with lunch and his needed insulin. His school day ended at one o'clock. I'll never forget the second year of his education, when he was promoted to first grade. He had been accustomed to staying only until one o'clock the year before and was quite indignant when he found out that he had to stay longer. After lunch that first day, he firmly said to the teacher's assistant, "Can I go home now? I'm sick of this damn place."

During my childhood years, I was either well protected or oblivious that there were problems in the world. A simple life meant a simple life. My parents' friends did not get divorced, my friends did not use drugs, people didn't get horrible diseases, and children didn't go hungry or unclothed. With the changes in the world, simplicity seems a thing of the past.

There are times in life when one gets wrapped up in one's everyday life and the time slips away. Once a moment is gone, it never comes back. The older I get, the more that realization is engrained in my mind. The last twelve years are nothing but memories now, with many more memories to look forward to as a school nurse. The sight of a small, innocent child, hanging in the balance, can in a heartbeat make you realize the fragility of life and how we should make every moment count.

A couple of weeks ago, after an illness, we all saw the Jesse that we previously knew at school: an energetic little boy who loves everyone and is as innocent as a little puppy. In fact, today he was proudly showing me the spare key to his mother's car. Hopefully, he won't decide to get in and start it up as he has done in the past.

Happy endings are wonderful. As with all of us, we won't know if Jesse will have a happy ending. Hopefully, it will be a long time before we know. I cherish the moments that he is healthy, and as a school nurse, I try to do my best to ensure the healthiest environment possible for all the children that I encounter every day in my job.

School nursing may sound simple. Simple is okay with me. If simple things in life make me feel like I did when I was a child, then I'm all in favor of simple. Here's the deal: I love my job. It makes me happy, it makes me sad, it makes me angry, it makes me love, and it makes me want to make a difference in the world, even if that difference is only through one child who, in return, has made such a dramatic imprint on my heart. And I wouldn't trade one day of all the memories of this job they call school nursing.

Kayla Mohling, BSN, RN
South Dakota

Triage

Having the knowledge, training, and ability to distinguish who will receive treatment first is a major asset in school nursing. Every school nurse must determine and make informed decisions based on her ability to differentiate between those in need of immediate medical care versus those that can wait. School nurses work in the "trenches," and for the benefit of all, are constantly adapting to the environment around them. Search through these stories written by school nurses to discover how they cope with these daily demands.

You Did What?

"I have noodles up my nose." The student states this as a matter of fact.

"How did you get noodles up your nose?" I ask.

"I laughed ... well, I kind of snorted when I laughed," he replies.

I have never seen this student before. He is not one of my frequent flyers, and he has informed me that he *can* breathe through his nose and he is supposed to be taking a test.

There are other students in my office. A student with a nosebleed, head hung over a trash can and dripping blood, explains that holding his nose doesn't work. He explains, "My mother tells me that it just has to bleed itself out." Another student sits quietly in a small off-to-the-side room and tells me that she "has" to talk with me. A pounding on my door stops all conversation. A student with her parent steps in. Evidently they are withdrawing and need the student's immunizations record "*now.*"

It isn't Monday, it isn't a full moon, and the line outside the door is growing. The paperwork is lined across my desk. Immunizations for the twenty-two new students are not even checked. The note that a care plan is needed for a new student with grand mal seizures is taped to my computer screen. Lodged on my bookshelf are the stacks of vision and hearing results from a mass screening the week before, still waiting to be filed and entered on the computer. The Medicaid paperwork is in a folder. I haven't read it yet, but a note on the front states that I need to get signatures. But right at this moment, I have a student with noodles up his nose that "needs to be taking a test."

I find the immunizations record for the student that is leaving and hand it to the mother. The line outside my door is getting longer as some of my frequent flyers and medication takers have arrived. No students with bleeding disorders, diabetes, or other high risks are seen. I get out my otoscope, and the student asks if this is going to hurt. I explain, "I am just looking for noodles." I suspect that I am in for a joke. Nope, noodles are there. Can't see them in his nose, but can see the ends dangling down from the back of the throat. The quiet student has now burst into tears. The nosebleed student is spitting large blobs of blood into the trash can. The quiet student tells me that she passes out when she sees blood. She is looking a little pale. Another student looks in the room and asks, "Can I borrow a female thing and use your bathroom?" The phone rings, and an administrator's assistant asks, "Do you have R. B.?" I hand the girl "the female thing," suggesting she use another bathroom. "Are any of you R. B.?" No R. B., but a student states that R. B. told their teacher that he was going to the bathroom to "puke." My noodle-nosed student asks if I am aware that he is missing his test. It is a typical day in the nurse's office.

My noodle-nosed student's mother is called. She will take him to the doctor. He will have to make up the test. The nosebleed student "gets" to hold his nose for twenty minutes, just to humor me to see if it might help. There is blood all over him and the trash can. R. B. has been located and was smoking in the parking lot, not puking. The quiet female student is pregnant; her parents do not know. An appointment is made for her with the "personal social counselor."

A teacher is trying to get my attention, but I am on the phone with a doctor taking medication orders for a student. A student accompanies the teacher. The student is pale. The trash can is too far away. He turns, and all eyes in the nurse's office are on him. Then vomit is flying through the air and lands on the wall, chair, and floor. A moment of silence, and then a call on the radio is made. "Clean-up needed on aisle three." Humor helps. Maintenance is on the way, and Captain Crunch will never look quite the same. I tell the student that he gets a 9.5 vomit score—pretty good. He smiles a little. It is still before lunch. I hope that they are not serving noodles.

I have approximately twelve hundred students at a high school. I usually see between thirty and seventy-five students per day. I have students that take daily medication, and a multitude of students that take "as-needed" medication. There are a number of medical concerns that have increased in my twenty years as a school nurse. More students are seen with life-threatening food/medication allergies, severe asthma, high blood pressure and pulse rates, cancer, pregnancy, Type II diabetes, depression, severe psychological and learning disorders, and seizure disorders. The list goes on and on.

More expectations are coming from schools and parents. These include needs for care plans and emergency plans. There are issues with students who are abusing alcohol and drugs, having sex, and self-mutilating. There are students who horse around and break glass windows and have altercations serious enough to warrant ambulance calls. There are normally four to nine ambulance calls each school year. There are parents who think I am the one responsible for all the staph and strep infections and that I am in charge of sanitizing all equipment throughout the school. I am never bored and enjoy working with this population of students.

Tamara Dorsett, BSN, RN
Kansas

MORE THAN TWENTY CENTS PER STUDENT

Coincidentally, at the time I was making the decision to wave my white flag of surrender to the stresses of hospital nursing, my local school district was launching what turned out to be its own little project. An innovative planner put together a grant-funded project that would place counselors and nurses in each school in the hopes that it would improve student attendance and performance. We started with the message, "Healthy kids are better learners," and began defining ourselves and building our program. After sixteen years, we are still unique in our area, since we use nurses to staff each building full-time rather than to manage and supervise unlicensed personnel at multiple school sites.

School nursing for me started in a tiny health room behind the school office. I had paper cups, glass thermometers, bottles of tincture of green soap, and a supply of one-inch adhesive bandage strips, most of which had been cut in half lengthwise to stretch out the supply. My annual budget amounted to about twenty cents per student, an amount considered generous compared to some schools. I longed for those expendable supplies I once casually sorted through or tossed out as "contaminated" in the local hospital pediatric treatment room. The single-use rolls of satin tape, bandages, and antiseptic swabs from IV start kits all were suddenly unreachable luxuries. I missed the hospital environmental services department, always there to "terminally clean" a potential infectious space and to fill idle moments dusting every surface in reach.

I quickly found that school nursing was working in the "trenches," adapting to limitations, and making small changes over time. I learned that diapering and colostomy care were possible on the office bathroom floor, while everyone in the office learned the value of an exhaust fan. School health records consisted of a small open-topped metal box of neatly creased five-by-nine cards that were expected to hold every health screening, special health concern, or physician contact note through the entire twelve years of a child's school life. We began creating more appropriate forms and documentation systems.

Once a full-time nurse was in place, a steady stream of visitors grew, and triage became the business of any given day. Thanks to a wise school secretary, who joyously handed over her "nurse job" to me, the one limiting factor to the flood of visitors was a small clinic pass each teacher was expected to send with the child, making them somewhat accountable for the decision to access the clinic. Somewhere along the way, I abandoned my plan to keep my foot in the door at the hospital as weekend staff. From the onset, I was exhausted, physically and emotionally. But I knew I was making a big difference for many children and their families.

Over time, school clinics in our district improved. We obtained locked storage systems for health records and medications. Today my clinic still has no restroom, but a sink was added as a small concession. Two years ago, we added a sophisticated electronic record system that generates what used to be tedious monthly data collections to document our productivity. A huge amount of other data and communications now go through that system as well, supporting our expanding school health programs. We organize asthma education programs each year for that 12 percent of our population who have asthma. Our district health services department has added teams of screeners for vision, hearing, and growth. Thanks to a well-organized professional volunteer corps, students receive dental screening and dental education each year. Since dental care is of particular need in our area, we apply dental fluoride varnish to a large segment of our population twice each year. Our nurses do case management health referrals to completion, facilitate access to health insurance, and assist families in finding primary physicians for "health care homes."

One of the most frustrating issues in school nursing for me is the reality that the nurse is the driving person in the school setting who is focused on health. What a difference from institutional health care! It is both rewarding and exhausting to be the only resource for problem solving daily health concerns of not only six hundred children, but seventy-five or so staff members. Education is *the* top priority business of the school, so health goals are secondary in every situation for teachers. Again, this is far different than in typical health professions. Teachers and administrators sometimes (as an afterthought, if at all) involve the nurse in planning for a child with special needs. I know I will need to learn, adapt, and remind teachers I am on their team.

For me, the reward of working in a school far outweighs the frustration. Health teaching has always been one of my very favorite parts of any kind of nursing. In the school, every minute of every day, every student contact is full of educational opportunities—teachable moments that can make a difference in a child's life. Validation for my effort comes through the thigh-high hug from a child in the supermarket and the wild screams of rock-star adoration from the backseat of the car next to me at a traffic signal. I have no doubt I make an impression in the lives of these youngsters. In return, they bring humor to my world daily. I recall a few weeks ago when my eight-year-old friend Miranda breezed in and out to make some quick adjustments to her insulin pump. As we clicked through her pump settings, another student watched in awe, asking a couple of questions that Miranda fielded in matter-of-fact style. The child's response was, "Wow! That was *sooo* cool!" But as Miranda and I walked out the door together beyond earshot, we laughed and shared a moment of connection as I whispered my thought, "You know what would be really cool … is if we could get your pancreas to do that."

I admit I feel at home with the repetition of these life situations: familiar sibling groups over the years, grandmothers who hold families together, and young alumni who return to visit, volunteer in some capacity, or bring a picture of their new baby. All of this reminds me that every encounter has a lasting impression. Just as lasting for me is the awareness of those subtle signs of a few of my "frequent flyers" with some classic behaviors of depression. I pray I will be tuned-in enough to recognize and intervene, to prevent what might otherwise become another teen suicide if I don't take action at the right time. Each day, whether joyous or particularly stressful, my intent is to let these six hundred students know they have value and potential.

Donna C. Maginness, BSN, RN
Missouri

Everything Hurts

As the school nurse for 239 fifth and sixth graders, I must be prepared for any emergency. Subjective information runs from, "I poked myself in the eye with my finger," to "My dog slept on my foot." Complaints vary from "paper cut" to "everything hurts." Children have been bumped with soccer balls, basketballs, badminton rackets, flutes, trombone cases, tone chimes, music stands, and lunch boxes. They fall at recess, on stairs, over backpacks, and from playground equipment. So far this year, I have had to assess forty-four sore throats, ninety headaches, and one hundred sixty stomachaches.

Objective data include temperatures up to 101.5 degrees, twenty-eight nosebleeds, one-millimeter cuts to seven-centimeter bruises, and a level of consciousness from alert/oriented to unresponsive with 911 called. Documentation over the past six months revealed that I have given forty-five cups of juice, forty-six cough drops, forty-seven tiny envelopes for teeth, one hundred ninety-two bandages, two hundred fifty-two cups of water, and three hundred twenty-nine ice packs. Three children take a daily medication. Fifteen students have asthma inhalers as needed. I have also handed out approximately three hundred boxes of tissues for classroom use.

Common assessments include the following: activity intolerance anxiety, fatigue, potential for infection, nausea, altered nutrition, pain, impaired skin integrity, and impaired social interaction. When a child is injured or ill, I often feel concerned and uneasy. The plan is to provide what is needed to return the scholar to class as soon as possible. Treatments can be simple, such as encouraging fluids, applying pressure to stop bleeding, or preventing infection. More complicated actions include calming anger, giving emotional support, or advising a multidisciplinary approach. Sometimes the child is sent home. Occasionally he/she is taken directly to the hospital by ambulance.

One bright student asked, "Wouldn't you rather be a doctor or veterinarian?" My answer was, "No, I always wanted to be a nurse."

Laura D. Fell, BSN, RN
Connecticut

Between Filling Out Reports

The day started with a delayed opening because the freshmen would be taking standardized tests. Marge, the high school head nurse, and I planned to use the quiet time to complete routine medical assessments that are due, and we are working on this when a teacher runs into our office and states, "There is a teacher down by the electric classroom." Marge grabs an emergency supply bag and the walkie-talkie and starts off down the hall. I lock up the office, grab the second emergency bag, and run to the site of the incident.

The teacher had been found unresponsive, lying on the ground in an awkward position. I glance at the pulse oximeter that Marge has placed on the victim's finger. It tells me we are not dealing with a cardiac event here. Something else is going on. Marge is in the process of assessing the victim's neurological status and performs a blood glucose test while I monitor blood pressure. Emergency services arrive. While they take over the scene, Marge interviews the people who found the victim and presents that information to the EMT.

I head to the administrative offices to find emergency contact information for the teacher. I give the information to the EMT and return to the health office. Marge stays behind, still talking to teachers and students at the scene. She will need whatever information they can give her in order to complete an incident report.

I find the students have started queuing up at the office door since the standardized testing is over. After seeing the students and entering their complaints and treatments into the computer, I look again at the report I am trying to do. Marge comes back and calls the emergency contact, explains what has happened, and has the hospital number ready for the family. Marge has also taken responsibility for the personal effects found at the scene and tells the family where they will be safely locked up.

I continue to see students while Marge returns to the scene in order to diagram the area for the accident report. She finds the teacher's students standing in the hall. Apparently, they had been sent to the wrong classroom by a note on the teacher's door and did not know what to do. Does someone really think adolescents are going to draw straws to see who is going to go to the office and report the double booking? No, they are going to continue to socialize with each other until someone in authority tells them what to do. Today that person is Marge. She finds out where the students need to be and sees that they get there before returning to the scene to collect the information necessary to complete the incident report.

I attend to students who have complaints that include headache, cramps, eye irritation, an itchy mosquito bite, and cuts and bruises. I administer prescribed medication fills in the morning and field various phone calls, including one from the parent of a student with hemophilia who wanted to let us know that the child is being treated for a bleed and is in a lot of pain but really wanted to come to school. Marge is busy trying to complete the incident report before leaving for a meeting at the middle school concerning one of the many medically complex students, whose safety she will be expected to be responsible for next year. I run to the cafe to pick up something to eat and take it back to the office. Marge never goes to lunch and always eats at her desk. I look longingly at the teachers in the cafe and think how nice it must be to have twenty minutes to eat away from the kids and socialize with your coworkers.

Marge finishes the incident report, sends a copy to the school superintendent, and heads for the middle school for the 1:30 p.m. meeting. Marge's contracted hours are 7:12 a.m. to 2:02 p.m. I smile and ask her if she is planning to stay for the entire meeting, knowing that she will not be compensated for her time. She smiles back and doesn't answer, but I know she will stay to the end. That's what nurses do. The meeting actually ended at 3:10 p.m.

Later in the day, one of the kids stops by to say that he didn't know that people my age could run so fast. I took it as a compliment.

The last student of the day has a nosebleed that won't quit but finally does. I look at what I wanted to accomplish today, the soon-to-be-overdue medical assessment. So far, I have the student's name, address, and birth date filled out. It's a start, and tomorrow is another day.

Ruthann Hatt, BSN, RN
Massachusetts

One Child at a Time

The school was a private K–12 school. The nursing clinic was a tiny room, more like a closet. We had four kindergarten-size chairs and a desk. I had an assistant who worked at the desk. I used the small chairs in my approach to patient treatment and consultation. I often sat on a tiny seat surrounded by children who were at eye level with me. It afforded a new view of life. I discovered that the eyes are indeed the lamp of the body. Troubled children have a faltering gaze, hungry children stare imploringly, and ill children … let's just say I learned to weed out the fakers.

I discovered a school nurse was part nurse, part mom, a friend replacement, a disciplinarian, someone who provided a safe haven, a counselor, a policewoman, a weapon and drug enforcement officer, a parent's last hope, a principal's thorn (or best bud), and if all is lost—someone to give a smile and a hug at the end of the day.

Through the years, I have been surprised at how many students wanted to hang around in the clinic with me and chat. At one point, when my son was in the upper grades, it was not unusual to find his friends joining him for lunch in the clinic. We had middle school and high school students who dropped by the clinic to chat or share confidences all day long. By that time, the clinic was larger, with three cots and many more chairs. However, the chairs remained kindergarten size. It was the way to keep face-to-face with little ones and make it just uncomfortable enough to discourage the older ones from using the clinic as a hideout.

During lunch we often had visitors. We all sat on tiny chairs, and kids shared stories or sometimes listened to my tall tales about life in the "olden days." Occasionally, someone would bring a guitar, and we had an impromptu songfest until either an emergency arrived or lunch ended. Sometimes I would serenade the captive audience and played my Celtic harp. I considered it harp therapy. The kids loved it.

Over time I earned the confidence of many kids who needed help to sort out adolescence. Once I was able to heal the wounds between two students who were on opposite sides. They would never be close friends again, but they came to the clinic at lunch period with groups of friends and sat in the little chairs while they listened to free-flowing conversation and relaxed with one another. They learned to respect each other. One lunch period, they were the only two who visited the clinic. Each pulled out a small chair and talked as they ate. Neither one would leave. They needed to outdo each other as they vied for my attention. But they were forced to listen to each other, and I hoped, to see each other in a new way. One of the principals came to the clinic on another mission during that lunch and quietly observed the scene. She stood transfixed for a moment. I have treasured the look that went between us as she turned and left the three of us sitting in small chairs listening to each other.

There was the suddenly single father who needed assistance with his kindergarten daughter. He was a well-intentioned father and an attentive dad. Now he was sole parent in charge.

Most of the time, illnesses or accidents were simple. However, I found that this was an arena with great teaching potential. Often parents did not recognize signs and symptoms or appropriate treatment for strep throat, chicken pox, scarlet fever, lice, scabies, flea bites, physical hygiene, oral hygiene, puberty changes, nutrition, impetigo or any number of skin infections, depression, cutting, and sexual abuse. The list is endless. Many parents were not sure when to keep their children at home. And there was the challenge to teach parents how to administer medication.

But there were situations that were serious. I had a few. After my first one, I realized how alone a school nurse was in an emergency. Effectiveness critically depended upon vital communication between the school nurse and the school staff. I worked on reasonable plans to assure that response to the playground or gym or wherever would not leave me isolated in an emergency. I was blessed with an office assistant who was my right hand, left hand, and usually my wings as well. I called to her for whatever I needed, and she was always there.

My first emergency was a fractured pelvis and femur from a fall during recess. I was as shaken as the child who suffered from the fall. I realized at once we could not move the child until EMS arrived. I was not prepared for this terrible accident. I relied upon basic first-aid practice and cried quietly when EMS arrived. The child did well and was able to play sports later in teen years. I then studied emergency care seriously and imagined scenarios in my mind and how best to respond.

My next event was an amputated finger. The child was in first grade. Fortunately, I knew her well due to her many visits. She was a frequent flyer. But we had trust. I was less shook that time. I remember most the dear teacher who trailed behind as she gingerly carried the digit in her hand. She gave it to my assistant and then collapsed. I am relieved to say the finger *was* successfully reattached.

The most unusual situation is also the one I recall in most detail. It happened to a child chewing on a pencil. She appeared in the clinic complaining of a sore throat. I examined her, and lo and behold: there was a round hole in her soft palate. The hole was the perfect size of an eraser on a number two pencil! The child confessed she pushed a pencil into her mouth by accident, and then pulled it out when she felt pain. There was no bleeding. I called EMS to ask for assistance. They arrived in less than five minutes. They cautioned me to expect bleeding and a compromised airway. Nothing of the sort ever happened. I was incredulous over the episode. However, we all have learned there are no "normal" injuries or average school nurse days.

Adventures continue even today. School nursing is a calling. It's not for everyone. I have to laugh now when I consider how I first felt about working with children. I can't believe what I might have missed. I have been a part of so many little miracles and so many lives. Even the experiences that brought pain and sorrow, I would not want to have missed. I am a better person for having the privilege of being a school nurse. I hear from students who graduated years ago. I love keeping in touch. I hear from teachers who have moved on as well. The school community is like a small village.

Sunny Kirkham, RN
Maine

"Tell Me ... I Can Take It!"

I had been a school nurse for about two years when one day a student walked into my office with a very serious expression on his face. He placed his hands on the edge of my desk, and leaning forward, he looked at me square in the eyes as I asked, "May I help you?"

He said, "I just swallowed my crayon!"

I quickly noted that his color was good and he was breathing and talking with ease. That was a good thing!

Then I thought, *How could this possibly happen?* I suddenly recalled watching a show on television where a man swallowed a sword, but remembered that was just a magic trick. I said, "What? How could you swallow a crayon?"

The boy responded, "I had it in my mouth and just swallowed it, by accident!"

"But how did you manage to do that and why?" I asked and then asked him how long the crayon was. The student held up his hand with his index finger and thumb about one and a half inches apart. I grabbed my penlight and told him to open his mouth so I could assess any injury to his soft palette or back of his throat. No bleeding or sign of injury was noted, and his gag reflex was intact.

The student had a desperately worried expression on his face. He said, "What's going to happen to me? Tell me, I can take it!"

Trying not to laugh, I told him that I would call his mom and tell her what happened. After I got off the phone, he asked again what would happen to him, so I pulled a body book off my bookshelf and opened it up to pictures of the alimentary system. I began showing him where the crayon would travel in his body. I explained that there might be a chance that the crayon would get stuck somewhere along the way out of his body, but not to worry because Mom was coming to take him to the doctor for an X-ray.

Mom arrived, and the boy showed her the book and said, "The crayon might get stuck inside me. What do you think, Mom?"

She turned to me, trying not to laugh, then looked back at him and said, "Let's see what the doctor says."

I told the boy to go to class and get his things. While he was gone, I told Mom that if the X-ray showed that her son was not in any danger of intestinal perforation, the doctor might take a wait-and-see approach.

The next day Mom called to tell me what happened when she took her son to the emergency room. She said that after her son had the X-ray and went back to the exam room, he asked the doctor, "What's going to happen to me? Tell me, I can take it." Then, both Mom and the doctor tried not to laugh.

The doctor sat beside the boy and said, "Son, I think you will be just fine. The crayon most likely will come out in a few days."

The boy's eyes got wide, and he asked, "How will I know if it came out?"

The doctor smiled and said, "That's easy. Each time you poop, it's your job to take these tongue blades and check the poop for your crayon."

Mom said that her son's mouth dropped open, his nose wrinkled, and he said, "You have got to be kidding!"

Shirley Rodriguez, BSN, RN, CSNP
Arizona

Counseling

The circumstances surrounding school nurse counseling are seemingly endless:

> ~A delighted little boy because his "new" and "dry" underpants have a magic marker "S" for Superman painted on by the school nurse
> ~Stressed out students who just want to talk to someone
> ~A stomachache cured in time for music class
> ~Telling a student to just sip, *not sit,* on a cup of tea!
> ~Getting lunch passes for students that otherwise would go hungry
> ~And all the other family, social, and medical counseling that a school nurse provides.

The school nurse is equivalent to the captain of a ship by guiding students, ensuring they have a safe journey. In addition, explore how a male school nurse counsels "surprised parents."

SPECIAL PASSES

September can be a very challenging time. Students are coming back from summer vacation. They are anxious and excited about the ensuing school year and have such high hopes and expectations. I, too, was nervous and unknowing of the expectations others had for me in my first years as a school nurse.

There is one LPN and myself who work in the wellness area. In this school of 980 students in grades seven through twelve, we see approximately sixty students a day. This includes those who are ill and those who need meds, as well as students who need emotional support or intervention.

As I was sitting in my office on that first day, a student came in and said that she was having some difficulty with stress. She thought it might be a good idea to come in and talk with me at some point. This young woman was very thin and exceptionally intelligent. She appeared to be nervous and shared little else except that she had some issues that would get in her way as the school year went on. She said she would come back and check with me later.

I will say that with 980 students at this point, my learning curve had not yet caught up with each student's needs. I immediately pulled her record to see what kind of issues she might need to address. This young lady frequently needed interventions.

She reappeared at my office door within the next hour requesting that she be able to sit with me to discuss a personal matter. We made an appointment, and she came in exactly on time, no hair out of place, perseverating on the day's events. We talked about several issues and came up with a plan for weekly discussion. I researched therapies with our school clinician, and we enrolled her in a skills group to build her self-help skills.

She continues to come in weekly; however, she now can use her skills to cope with most situations that arise. She is now looking forward to school and what education can do for her future goals. She has a vision to finish school and go on to higher learning. I do believe that had the circumstances been different and without support systems to assist her, she would not have flourished and there would have been a very different outcome.

My second school story involves about twenty students. Throughout the school year, my nurse had been observing an influx of students in the wellness center at breakfast and lunch times. We both began exploring why it was at these times that students would come to our area and tend to hang around. The students seemed to be looking for something that they were not asking for. Then one of our seventh-grade students came in and revealed that not only her family, but many families that she and her family knew, had lost their qualification for free and reduced-cost meals. Both of their parents were now working, but they made too much money to qualify anymore for the food program. These students were not being provided with lunch money. Their families could also not afford to buy additional lunch foods to give these students to carry with them. In fact, for many of these families, just paying for fuel oil or gas to get to work had become a priority.

As we all know, when students don't eat, they are unable to learn. My nursing counterpart and I came up with a plan called "the golden pass" and established a fund to pay for it. This entitled those students to come in and retrieve a pass that allowed them to eat for free. We reviewed the students that were taking advantage of this and found that some of them were eligible to apply under a different program; we asked the school social worker to set it up for them. We made these efforts so all of our students could always have breakfast and lunch.

Wanda Bouvier, RNC
Vermont

SUPER SOLUTION

Let me share with you one of the most hilarious moments in my career; it involves an adorable little boy with the most beautiful smile that covered his whole face. One day, fairly early in the school year, at the busy noontime lunch and recess hour, he was brought into my office having had an "accident" out on the playground. He did not have that beautiful smile on his face, but was trying very hard to hold back his tears. A cursory glance showed me a telltale wet area on the front of his pants. Although the office was crowded with other students, things were under control, so I immediately led him into the bathroom (which fortunately was part of my office). I soothed his anxieties and assured him I would attempt to contact his mother to have her bring a change of clothes. However, as was the case a great deal of the time, she was a working parent who was unable to leave her job just to bring him in a change of clothes.

Since this was a common problem in my school, I had worked with the PTA to purchase underwear and socks in a variety of colors and sizes for both boys and girls. I also had gathered used pants, tops, sneakers, and so on, which parents had given me in various sizes. These were all kept in a dresser and shelves that I had set up in the bathroom. Actually, it was a joke in my school that my bathroom was almost as big as my whole office. So I got together (with what I thought was his input) dry underwear, socks, pants, and sneakers. His top was not wet and therefore did not need to be changed. I asked him if he could handle changing those items himself, and he assured me he could. When he was finished, he was to put his wet clothes into a plastic bag I had given him; he was then to come back out of the bathroom and let me know he was ready to go back to class.

Back in the office, I got busy handing out daily meds and managing several other incidents that needed handling. Suddenly there was some commotion among some students in the office, as well as some students who had been passing my office in the hallway.

When I turned around and looked, there was my little friend standing totally and absolutely naked, with the strangest expression on his face. He looked up at me and said, "I can't wear those underpants because they don't have Superman on them, and I only wear Superman underwear."

I quickly got him back into the bathroom and tapped some ingenuity that only fellow school nurses could understand. I got some red and black permanent markers and drew the Superman logo on the underpants with a big "S" as best as I could remember it. It was sufficient to please him, and the great big smile came back to his face. His day was made, and mine was too.

Patricia Marsh-Thorell, BSN, RN
New Hampshire

THE STOMACHACHE

Many kids complain of stomachaches. This seems to be the physiological ailment a child has when he or she is bored, hungry, over-full, sad, constipated, or just missing mom. Stomachaches can be the most difficult to assess to determine if the student needs to be seen by a doctor, is ill enough to go home, or can stay at school.

On one occasion, a little girl with sad eyes hung her head when she came to my nurse's clinic. She had tears running down her face, and upon questioning, she reported having a "bad" stomachache and that she wanted Mommy. I did an assessment that found no elevated temperature and no signs of appendicitis or other abdominal distress. However, I was unable to console her. I suggested to her that she lie down for a while on my cot and rest. This would enable me to observe her.

After just a few minutes, she jumped up with a smile on her face and said, "Teacher said to be back by ten, 'cause we have music." Off she went skipping down the hall and back to her class. I would like to think that it was my good care that cured her, but I think it was the allure of her music class instead.

Gloria Jean Reynolds, BSN, RN, CSN
Illinois

Everything Isn't Always What I Hear

I had one of my "frequent flyers" come to the clinic one day last fall. The girl, a senior, complained that she was having a hard time urinating. Since I had seen her so much over the last three years and I was very familiar with her parents, I didn't hesitate to inform them. I have had numerous conversations with her parents, so I was well aware of the fact that they were very big advocates of homeopathic medication. I called the mom to inform her of her daughter's newest affliction. After hearing my assessment of the situation, Mom said, "Have her sit on a cup of warm water." I politely acknowledged her response and passed the advice on to her daughter, who was waiting in the clinic. The student quickly said, "I have done some weird things, but I *refuse* to sit on a cup of warm water!" When I heard her repeat what I thought I had heard, I started laughing so hard I cried! I realized my mistake in hearing. Her mom intended her to "sip," not "sit," on a cup of warm water.

Patti J. Twaddle, RN
Tennessee

THE LITTLE BOY AND HIS SHOES

For most kids, getting ready for a new school year includes a trip to the store for new school supplies, new clothes, and new shoes. Yet, for some this is not so. Their families struggle to get by, and these children have clothes and shoes that have already seen their better days or are hand-me-downs at best. As a school nurse, my job includes many different aspects. As the school year starts, I am busy collecting physicals, setting up medication schedules, checking medical conditions, and doing a host of other things.

One of the jobs I have taken on is "checking for shoes," for lack of a better term. In my community, we are fortunate to have some organizations that donate time and money to help children in different ways. One such organization donates shoes for those children who wouldn't otherwise have a new pair. Once a year, I make a list and get a bus that takes the students to the local discount shoe store.

I remember one year in particular. There was a little boy who was seven years old. He was very quiet. I gave him a permission slip and told him to have his parent sign the form and return it to me. "I'm going to get new shoes!" he exclaimed.

He told his teachers about his upcoming trip. Every day he stopped by the clinic to be sure the trip was still on. On the day of the trip, he lined up with the other students, eager to be on his way. At the store, the clerk measured him for his size, and then we went through the racks of shoes. He picked out a pair of white lace-up running shoes. When he put them on, he beamed. I told him he could wear them back to school if he liked. He said he would only wear them at school and wanted to wear his old shoes to and from school so that the new ones would not get dirty.

When he returned to his classroom, he carefully put his new shoes back on and showed them to all the other students and his teachers. He wrote a story about his trip to the store, and then he came to the clinic with a note for me. It was a thank you. When I looked at him after reading the note, I could see that his new white shoes didn't shine near as much as his big happy smile.

Gloria Jean Reynolds, BSN, RN, CSN
Illinois

Yes, the Nurse Is Here ...
You're Looking at Him

When I became a school nurse more than halfway through my nursing career, the first thing that struck me was the walk from my car to my office: about twenty feet from the parking lot to the clinic door. No parking garage. No parking fee. No unsecured employee parking three blocks away in a sketchy neighborhood, like every other nursing job I'd ever had in a dozen hospitals over twenty years.

It made me think of what one of my mentors had said when I was still a green-smocked student: "Day shift, street clothes, and a good parking space, Robert. That's the key to being happy in nursing."

To add to my good fortune, I got the Cadillac of school clinics. Most clinics in my district are afterthoughts, converted broom closets and overhauled volleyball storage rooms, but I got an actual classroom with a sink, refrigerator, computer, printer, fax machine, and a private bathroom.

This is it, I determined that first morning. *This is the job I'm going to do until I retire or die, whichever comes first.* Note that I made this definitive declaration without having yet seen a single student. In case you're wondering, yes, years later, I still feel exactly the same way. I found my niche. I solved the riddle of "What do I wanna be when I grow up?"

As a child, being a nurse never crossed my mind. At age forty-four, being a school nurse is all I can imagine doing. Unless, by some remote chance, the original plan to be a Beatle or Superman works out.

No situation is ideal, though. Even people who review cruise ships for a living get tired of pineapple juice and the song "Hot, Hot, Hot." There are aspects of the job that grow tedious, such as relaying empathy. Not the empathy itself—as I genuinely feel bad for every red-faced, bleary-eyed child that stumbles in either the pre- or post-stage of vomiting—but the expression of emotion. There are officially only forty-seven ways to convey your sympathy in the vomiting circumstances. I won't list them all, but trust me, between "Oh, you poor thing!" and "Ye gads, what did you eat?", there are *exactly* forty-seven variations. I've counted them.

Vomit etiquette isn't the only aspect of the school nursing role that chafes, however. There's a more immediately obvious one that involves my having an Adam's apple and facial hair. I'm talking about being a guy and a school nurse. A *male* school nurse.

Take a second. Repeat that phrase in your head. Now, what was the first thought you conjured? Be honest; I can take it. In the best-case scenario, you pictured a stranger talking to your child, and your next thought was to intervene—and for a parent, that's a completely reasonable reflex. If I'd just said "school nurse," you would have been allowed to imagine a lovely blond woman in a crisp white uniform with a cap patting your little nipper's head, and it would fill you with relief and appreciation.

Instead, you pictured something akin to when your children wander too far from you at the fair and you don't like the way the carnie who runs the Tilt-a-Whirl is looking at them. Your first impression may have been more visceral and fearful. And that is what I encounter a dozen times a day.

So how do I convince small kids and their parents that I can be trusted? Besides by being a female? I mean, I could go that route, but I don't think in the end it would help all that much, and my wife would probably object.

I practice the age-old deflection of humor. Kids nowadays have even shorter attention spans than we did growing up, thanks to five hundred channels and strobe-lit handheld video games. In the world we've created, kids generally give you five seconds before they completely tune you out. It's easy to both get a child's attention and disarm their apprehension by setting them at ease with a joke. It's easier than with adults, who often have had their sense of humor surgically removed along with their appendix and their capacity for joy.

I've never stood up in front of a fake brick wall on open mike night, but I like to think I know my way around the funny. The average third grader finds me hysterical. Examples, you ask? Here are some greatest hits I'll pass onto you at no extra cost.

Ask me how tall I am, and I'll tell you six foot four, give or take a foot. Tell me that nurses are supposed to be girls, and I'll slap my forehead and say, "So, that's why my mom keeps mailing me training bras!"

* * *

When I meet any of the elementary-age children I've treated over two decades, their anxious eyes are as wide as saucers. "So," I will always begin, "… what kind of car do you drive?"

Stunned surprise eventually gives way to a sideways grin and the same incredulous reply each time: "I don't have a car."

"Oh. You make your spouse drive?"

* * *

A lunch box upends across the floor of my clinic, and inexplicably, a hundred screws and nails splay out. "Did Bob Vila pack your lunch today?"

* * *

One of my diabetic kids has a higher-than-average blood sugar: "I don't care what they say on TV; pancake syrup is not an acceptable mouthwash."

* * *

"Take your medicine, please."
"No."
"What did the skeleton order when he went to a bar?"
"I don't know, what?"
"I'll tell you after you take your Ritalin."
"Fine! There, I took it. What's the answer?"
"Bartender, I'll have a beer and a mop."

* * *

These exchanges and a million more like them have been my best way to warm up to kids who needed my help but were afraid to trust a stranger, either because their mother wisely told them not to or because, tragically, the world has taught them they shouldn't. When parents meet me at PTA and remind me of the jokes their children repeat to them at home prefaced by "Mom, you have to hear what Mr. Robert said," that's pretty cool.

This is the point where I should probably say something about laughter being the best medicine, but I think the *Saturday Evening Post* went out of business, didn't it? So, I'll spare you the bromide and say that a child who is laughing barely notices an old Band-Aid being pulled off, and I'll leave it at that.

Robert D. Naugle, AND, BFA
South Carolina

A Mighty Purpose

One day a student came to my office with pain in his stomach. He said a door had swung and hit him in the stomach. His head ached as well. I took his temperature. Knowing he had a chronic disease, I also knew pain and fever could be serious signs of a crisis situation. He had a low-grade temperature of 99.8 degrees. I thought to myself that if his temp climbed over 100 degrees, coupled with the pain he had, he would need an ER visit. I gave him fluids and called his mom to tell her I was watching him closely and would keep her informed. His mom apprised me of the home situation.

I sat down with the student and told him that I knew he couldn't possibly like what was going on in his home. I explained that it was possible for there to be peace between him and his mom and love could be expressed between them. He didn't talk or look at me. Speaking as a mom, I told him that our children are our heart. I choked up when I said that I can disagree with my husband, but when it came to my children, arguing was devastating. He looked at me with tears streaming down his face. He sobbed and listened while I spoke. I painted the picture of what a happy family could look like. After awhile, I took his temperature again. It had gone down to 98.6 degrees. His head and stomach were better, and he returned to class.

I relayed this to his mom, who was relieved and appreciative. I also recommended therapy to resolve hurts that are in the past but affecting him now—"stuck feelings." She later reported to me that that night, he listened, and she was able to return his privileges. They were happier. His affect changed in school; he looked calm and became friendlier. Things just got better and better at home. I did, however, recommend again that he speak to a counselor to make sure the past does not affect his relationships in the future. I am privileged to have made a difference for him and his family.

I came in early one Monday morning to find a student leaning over a garbage pail, actively sick to her stomach. I approached her and did several automatic assessments, feeling her head for skin temperature, color, and moisture for evidence of fever. I walked her to my office and observed her pain and energy level. There I took her temperature, blood pressure, and pulse, the vital signs reflecting the health of her vital organs. I knew she was not in any danger at that point. Taking a history, I was able to clear that there were no health problems in the last twenty-four hours. I then asked about stresses in her life, including if her homework were done and if she was prepared for the day. She said no. I asked her if she thought this was bothering her. Nonverbal, she nodded her head yes. I took out a computer and gave her the time to complete the homework. As she started to write the answers, I gave her juice and crackers, with no resulting stomach upset. She needed to eat to raise her energy level. With her physical health restored and homework done, she could join her class and complete the rest of the school day. I spoke with her mother and reinforced how important it was to have her come to school prepared.

With my nursing education and personal training in communication and effectiveness, I facilitate an increase in instruction time and contribute to the academic progress of the student. In turn, academic success inspires more success—giving children the confidence to go forward. What a privilege it is to be a school nurse!

School nurses also have an opportunity to work on a team in the education setting. Nursing is a perfect partner with social work, teaching, and administration. I contribute my part along with a team of teachers and administrators who are as passionate as I am. The only way other disciplines will truly understand the value of nursing judgment is by my describing what I do and why. It is up to me to influence what people know and understand about school nursing. If I stop and look and value what I do, others will understand and value my role as well.

I come in early and leave late. I do planning, research, and report writing on weekends so I can spend time while I am in the school caring for the students. During the day, my work is interrupted too frequently for me to be able to think deeply on the job for more than three minutes at a time! Honestly, I experience sheer joy in seeing the students' progress. I know I am doing what I was put on the earth to do.

Laurie Rufolo, MSN, RN
New Jersey

The Proper Care and Feeding
of a School Nurse

I have often felt blessed to have studied both nursing and counseling. It is as if I have found an "owner's manual" of how the body and mind work. I have wondered how people live life without this vital information.

After working for over twenty years as both a critical care nurse in a hospital and as a counselor in private practice, I felt called to the career of school nurse. Although I have had extensive training and study, each day in the school setting brings its own challenges, worries, and celebrations.

Throughout the years of my training, I have been blessed with many wonderful teachers, who have given me very sound advice. One teacher, in particular, taught me that "We can only take our students as far as we have gone ourselves." I have taken this to mean that if I want to help others to fully achieve their potential physically, mentally, emotionally, and spiritually, then it is essential that I apply self-effort to do the same for myself.

I believe that a school nurse has to be on top of her game at all times and always be prepared should an emergency arise. My office is often a combination of the emergency room (where I mend injuries and illnesses) and the department of health (where I make sure all the immunizations, health screenings, and other requirements are up-to-date).

I am continuously working to keep my light shining brightly from the moment I wake up in the morning to the moment I go to sleep at night. My day actually starts with the night before as I focus on my own fitness goals: eating healthy and getting plenty of sleep so that my mind is sharp and my body is strong to face the challenges of the day. When I awake, I meditate to calm my mind and exercise to get my body moving in high gear, taking in a healthy dose of oxygen. I shower and have a healthy breakfast, keeping in mind I can only preach what I practice. I also know that I have to be in tip-top shape because I want to be ready for whatever challenges I will be facing that day.

When I walk into school, my body feels good, my head is clear, and I am in a cheerful mood as I greet faculty, support staff, and students with, "Hey, how are you, what's up?" When I see a sad face or a new bandage, I register that for a later conversation in private. I keep in mind that it is I whom they turn to in their hour of need, and it is me they tell their hidden health secrets to. I do not take this lightly. I keep this information confidential, and I keep myself welcoming all, so that they will feel safe in my presence.

Many students come in the morning with complaints of being tired or dizzy or having stomach or headaches. They are used to my standard question, "Did you have breakfast this morning?" Anticipating the answer no, I have filled my cabinets with granola bars and cereal. I often get smiles, and occasionally students will proudly proclaim, after many repeated visits, that they indeed remembered to have breakfast that morning and they are adding more protein into their diet, which actually helps them feel more energy.

Being a school nurse feels like being the "school Mom," with over a thousand kids of different ages. Being the school nurse means being the "calm in the storm," while making sharp clinical decisions when a student is having a seizure, has no blood pressure, has cut three-fourths of his finger off, has overdosed on a bunch of pills, or is having an allergic reaction. It is about thinking quickly on your feet, stabilizing the student, getting the student to safety, and keeping everyone calm during the process.

There will be a student running in the office with a trail of blood behind him, having just cut his finger in cooking class. While putting direct pressure on the wound to stop the bleeding, I assess his anxiety level and reassure him. Once the bleeding has stopped, I check to see when he had his last tetanus shot, and I call the mom: "Mrs. So-and-So, this is the school nurse... Everything is okay. I want to let you know I have So-and-So here. He's okay, but he cut his finger. It looks like he may need stitches, but the bleeding has stopped. Would you like to talk to him? Be careful driving... He's okay, he is in good hands, and his tetanus shot is up-to-date."

I have had over a hundred conversations with a female student who was acting out in different ways as she experienced the fears of adapting to a new environment. I kept encouraging her to believe in herself; and one day, she came into my office saying, "Just wanted you to know, Ms. A., you are right... I am getting stronger. I am seeing myself change in a positive way, and it is amazing. I can't believe it!" Her behavior and grades are improving. It has truly been a gift to witness her growth in confidence.

Patricia H. Allocca, LCSW, RN, CSN
New Jersey

Evaluation

One must marvel at the skill school nurses have for the development and implementation of individualized health care assessments and management plans for medically fragile children attending school. Additionally, in order for the regular school population to receive medical care, documentation is also required. Throughout the day, the school nurse is constantly evaluating every child that comes into the medical office, regardless of the reason for the visit. Evaluation is an ongoing occurrence, and reading this chapter's stories is one way of learning the process.

A "Plum" of a Job

Jack Horner
Little Jack Horner
Sat in the corner,
Eating his Christmas pie;
He stuck in his thumb,
And pulled out a plum,
And said, "What a good boy am I!"
Anonymous English author

I recently had the opportunity to testify before the state senate health care committee regarding the state of school nursing. One of the comments from a senator was: "School nursing, what a plum of a job." As I heard these words, I was struck with many emotions, from indignation to sadness to surprise.

Initially, I felt offended by the remark. How could someone who has not walked in my shoes say I have an easy job? School nurses have a very challenging and sometime precarious profession. Challenging due to the nature of the environment in which we work, and precarious because of the balance we must maintain between nurse/school, nurse/parent, and nurse/child. This is beginning to be recognized by state boards of nursing around the nation, as many are issuing position statements and supporting briefs describing the specialized role of the school nurse.

School nurses work in an educational setting and must learn how to translate nursing language into educator language. For example, nursing assessments become "present levels of performance." Nursing outcomes become "short-term goals and objectives." School nurses are responsible for translating complicated medical diagnoses and plans into language that parents and teachers understand. We train individuals with little or no medical background on how to perform complex medical procedures for children in the school environment, and this process is often chaotic and unpredictable. We are the liaison between teachers and families when children with chronic or acute medical conditions attend our schools. School nurses can be compared to preventive medicine: if we are doing our jobs correctly, no one will notice because there are no negative outcomes.

I was also saddened by the remark because it proves the point that the general public does not understand what school nurses do. They still think we sit at a desk in a white uniform and put Band-Aids on scraped knees, take temperatures, and give reassuring hugs to little ones. School nurses deal with so much more. The number of children coming to school with chronic health conditions, such as asthma, diabetes, epilepsy, and anaphylaxis, continues to rise at staggering rates. These children require individual health assessments and management plans for making school a safe place for them. Due to the unparalleled advances in medical science in the last several decades, children who would not have survived birth or infancy are now coming to school. School nurses advocate for these students' inclusion in the educational setting and are responsible for providing medical services that will keep them healthy and alive at school.

Gone are the days of the one- or two-room schoolhouses, and gone are the days of the schools with only one hundred or two hundred students. Today, school districts are developing large, "super" schools, where several schools or school programs are housed together. They are using community workplaces for education in an effort to meet the needs of evolving student populations. Yes, school environments have changed dramatically in the past few decades, as have the needs—both educational and medical—of the students.

The final reaction I had to the remarks made by the senator was surprise. However, once I took time to adequately think it through, I agree that school nursing is a "plum" of a job. We use our nursing skills and knowledge of assessment, planning, intervention, and evaluation every day. We work with a team of professionals who are committed to providing the very best education possible for children. We see families in the "real world," not the artificial environment of the hospital or clinic. Because of this, we can effect positive changes in the lives of our patients much more readily than nurses in other settings. School nurses can make a difference in the lives of children. What better job could there be?

Nina R. Fekaris, MS, BSN, RN, NCSN
Oregon

Every Student Deserves a School Nurse

School nursing involves more than putting on Band-Aids. It consists of taking care of students who have multiple medical problems and making sure that students are in the safest learning environment. Is the school nurse available to take care of the student in the event of an asthma attack? Is the school nurse available to give medications? If not, it is the school secretary or the school principal who gives the medications and treats the student having an asthma attack. What about the students who require certain procedures, such as tube feedings and catheterizations? Again, it's not always the school nurse. We have to train unlicensed personnel to perform these procedures safely, as well as teach them what complications to look for and what to do in an emergency. In these cases, the development of a health care plan (IHP) is also required, and everyone who is involved with the student (including the bus driver) must have a copy, understand the information, and agree to follow the instructions. In my school, approximately one-third of the students have a medical diagnosis requiring a health care plan. Multiply this by the number of schools the nurses are responsible for covering—usually three or four schools.

During the middle of the week, we conduct mandated team vision and hearing testing. This only leaves nurses two days during the week to go to three or four schools. Add in all of the IEP's for which the nurse is required to create a health care plan, and then multiply that times the number of schools the nurse has. How well would you do your job if you only were able to be in your office one half day a week and be expected to "catch up" on a week's worth of work in that half day?

Nurses are not the top priority in the school system. There is not a nurse in every school! Our state mandates that the nurse-to-student ratio is 1:1,500. My caseload is the lightest in our system. I have two schools, with about one thousand students. I am also acting as the "unofficial" assistant head nurse. My colleagues have anywhere from fifteen hundred to two thousand plus students.

Nurses not only medically take care of students, but we also educate students about their health. We teach them about different things, such as basic hygiene and what is going on with their bodies. We educate them about diseases and immunizations. We strive hard to promote healthy students who are up-to-date on the immunizations recommended by the Centers for Disease Control. Explaining a disease, its transmission, and what can be done to prevent it makes the student understand why this is so important.

I am one of the lucky school nurses. I have an office where I can get my work done. By no means is it perfect. One of my offices is actually a closet. The other is a classroom, which I share with special education staff, the police officer, and the janitors. Great confidentiality! Some of my colleagues don't have an office. One of our nurses actually was given the back of a classroom where the teacher is teaching a class! Try and talk to a student who comes to you for advice about the possibility of pregnancy while you are in the back of a classroom. We have done hearing screenings in the halls, bathrooms, and stairwells. Basically, we do the best we can with the resources we have available.

It is time we give our students what they deserve ... a nurse in every school!

Verna Thompson, BSN, RN
Louisiana

Outside the Gym Closet

Choosing nursing as a career has provided me opportunities to meet my professional as well as personal needs for over twenty years. One of those opportunities almost slipped past me in the course of a side-yard conversation. The headmaster of a local private school asked me if I would be interested in a school nurse position opening up at his school. A dozen thoughts went through my mind, such as: low pay, poor benefits, and little professional stimulation. I pictured myself being placed in a small room shuffling immunization records most of the day. I looked down to the ground to avoid any trace of "Are you kidding me?" showing up in my face, but then I quickly remembered a life lesson I had once learned about burning bridges. I agreed to an interview, and years later, I continue to be amazed at the joys and professional fulfillment I experience as this school's nurse.

My experience is due, in large part, to the reality that my employer recognizes what roles an RN can play in the school setting. I not only have the materials necessary to do my job, but I also have the freedom to explore the many facets of school nursing. This has best been exemplified by the work I have done as the administrative representative on our health and safety committees.

The health committee, in particular, is made up of some very passionate mothers who have accepted the charge from our headmaster to develop and implement an annual "Respect Your Body" week. The first year we focused on nutrition. The committee identified volunteers to set up a sample food line for our secondary students following an assembly on eating healthy. Closeted health-food gurus came out in full force! These mothers handed out samples of every type of health food imaginable, and our students obliged them with such a willingness to try new foods that we knew we struck gold. Three years later, we continue this annual tradition.

In addition, recently we joined forces with Garden of Life, a national health-food company, in a health initiative for interested staff and families of our students. Approximately fifty families of students and staff participated in the full twelve weeks of the program, which provided nutritional education and support, and there are current plans to provide some of these opportunities throughout the school year. In working closely with the administration and families of our students, my role has expanded in the program's impact. It has been exciting to hear back from the students and faculty about the lifestyle changes their families have made. For some, it was the first real success they had ever experienced in making such dramatic changes.

Looking back on that fateful day seven years ago, I can say I am proud to be counted among the thousands of school nurses across America. Although I do have a small office (the old gym closet) and mounds of health records, I spend little time in there taking care of immunization records. I hope that in the future, I will hear that I am not an anomaly in my field of practice. Perhaps more and more administrators, as well as politicians, will recognize the impact school nursing can have on the health of the upcoming generations and provide the means to expand our roles.

Dorothy Patrock, MS, RN, SANE-A
Oklahoma

GRATEFUL TO SERVE

I greet you today from a rural community, where I work as the school nurse in a setting with approximately eight hundred students. The students who attend our school come from varied economic levels and different social and family backgrounds.

My six years of school nursing follows a long and diverse career path. I really believe that my position at this school and this place in time was determined, in part, by divine guidance. I am truly grateful to be here to share my experience and offer what guidance and support that I can to the students. Also, I have found that my age has aided me in decision making with a bit of insight in helping me to understand the problems of today's youth.

In addition to my already heavy workload, the added challenge that I am facing this year is to complete, by the end of the school year, the assessment documentation that is now required regarding the care given to each student. With all the mandated rules and regulations, plus emergencies, chronic illnesses, conferences with parents for community services, counseling students, giving out medications, caring for medically fragile students, and the frequent flyers that come into my office, the end of the school day is upon me, and I have run out of time to finish my work.

The staff and I recognize the numerous problems that this generation of youth is confronted with daily. We work diligently toward providing the physical, emotional, and educational needs necessary to help them become productive future citizens.

I love my job, and I strive to do my best, each and every day, even though at times it seems almost impossible to function due to all the stress. My aim is to help however I can to direct these students on the right path to becoming happy and healthy individuals. I am grateful for the opportunity to serve these students, and I would not dream of changing my job.

Carol Ray, LPN
Alabama

The Acorn and the Tree

I rather naively began my career as a school nurse more than fifteen years ago. I thought that I would just do this job for a few years while my three daughters were finishing high school, as my schedule matched theirs. What better nursing job could there be with vacations, weekends off, and the most glorious part: two months off in the summer. All of this, and an amazing salary of $15,000 per year! How hard could this be?

I have definitely lost my innocence. The changes that have taken place in the last fifteen years have been astounding. I'm sure they are indicative of society as a whole and not just related to changes in the children of today. I have witnessed more anger (especially in girls) being acted upon, with violent fights and sometimes with extremely abusive and vulgar language directed at me. There have been times that I have been afraid for my own safety. The smallest incident today can spark a barrage of vulgarity and obnoxious behavior from a fourteen-year-old. If I tell a student that they do not show severe enough symptoms to send them home for a day, I'm generally seen as a "mean" nurse. I have been told that I should go get a degree in nursing, as I don't know what I'm talking about; parents have been disrespectful enough to quote that belief to me.

I will never forget the best advice I have received since I began this career. It came from my first principal, who said, "Just remember, the acorn doesn't fall too far from the tree." I can't tell you how many times I have quoted that to myself over the years. It sure helps to keep everything in perspective. From poverty to teenage pregnancies, to disrespect, hypochondria, poor attendance, and substance abuse, the teenager most likely is just modeling behavior that has been a part of their life since birth.

A young boy complaining of a stomachache came into the clinic a few years ago. I thought he was trying to avoid class but sat him down to talk to him. He became very sad and burst into tears. Through his sobs, he finally confided that he had been having problems at home. We were able to make the social services calls and end his misery. That young man now is one of our top-notch citizens. Nothing compares to the satisfaction of helping students change a troubled situation into something positive.

Another change this career has brought to my life is the stripping away of prejudices. We all have our opinions formed on teenage pregnancies and how bad this is for society. I have since learned that this is a very "curable disease" and many young moms can become very successful. I had a pregnant student a few years ago who has now accomplished a four-year college degree, become a professional businesswoman, and is obtaining her master's degree.

I have also learned the lessons of not coddling the students, nor letting them use their aches and pains as reasons to shirk responsibilities. Physical education class is not one of the popular classes among teenage girls. I love the opportunity to teach them that menstrual cramps occur once a month and we have to learn how to cope with them. Colds and headaches happen to everyone, and taking pain relievers really does work. I try to teach that in the real world, where you have a job, your employer expects you to come to work even though you are not in the most perfect state of health. We can still function with some aches and pains.

Health insurance programs have gone through many changes, and this is making my job more challenging each year. Many of the families in my community are considered "the working poor"; they have jobs that don't provide insurance, and yet they fall below the income level required for Medicaid. This makes it difficult to obtain treatment for the kids, who have so many recurring illnesses. The same can be said for dental health.

I have seen an increase in illegal drug use in the past few years. Many school districts have been hit hard with the misuse of prescription drugs. Hydrocodone has been the number one "drug of choice" this year. I have been increasingly alarmed at the young age that the kids are streetwise to these types of drugs. The long-term side effects of these drugs are still being determined, but we know that the liver and kidneys can be damaged with the use of such drugs. The kids state boredom, stress, and self-medication as the reasons why they try these drugs.

Physical activity in teens has decreased sharply since I began my career. We have to beg the kids to play sports. This has led to the increase in our number of obese teens. They prefer to sit in front of their computers and send instant messages to their friends. They have a wealth of info at their fingertips. Chat rooms are a world of their own, and some of them can be very scary. The federal government is now on board with the issue of teen obesity.

I have contemplated the question, "If you had it to do over again, would you have stayed in school nursing this long?" I can say yes; it has been a rewarding nursing career, but it is not for the person with low self-esteem or low self-confidence. School nursing has changed me in many ways and has made me into a better person. Every nurse begins their career with the desire to help people and make a difference. At the end of mine, I can say that this has been what has kept me motivated.

Eunice Arendt, RN
New York

SWINE FLU

Swine flu, the H1N1 virus, made the national news in the winter of 2009, with lots of media frenzy and speculation. With lots of rumors and suspicions about possible cases in the county, school nurses as well as the county health department began implementing our crisis plan in preparation for an outbreak. The precautions in the school setting included recording and tracking trends in flu symptoms for all children and adults that came to the school clinic. Teachers and staff in the school were encouraged to practice good hand washing and to instruct their students to do the same. We had a newsletter sent home with a brief explanation about swine flu, as well as precautions to take. For example, we gave parents a list of symptoms that their children might exhibit that would warrant keeping them home from school.

In April 2009, our preparation, tracking, and education came into play as the first case of swine flu was confirmed in the school district. I was asked to assist the county health department school liaison as the investigation began at the elementary school. Upon our arrival to the school campus, we were met at the entrance by media trucks, reporters, and parents. Our job at the school was to collect data, take statements, and identify who was at risk. The staff and administration at the elementary school were very helpful and willing to provide any assistance and documentation we needed. With the implementation of our new school health computer database, I was able to pull information about students' visits to the clinic and health history in order to identify students at risk for contracting the swine flu. Letters were sent home daily to parents updating them on the situation. Staff and administration met daily to receive updates and to reinforce important precautions to use in the school to prevent any further cases.

Under the guidance of the Centers for Disease Control and the health department, the elementary school was closed for three school days in order to clean the campus and decrease the chances of spreading swine flu from student to student. There were a total of three confirmed cases among the students, and all three did recover from the illness.

This highly publicized outbreak brought more awareness to the need for health education and medical information in the schools. School nurses, with their information and expertise, were vital to parents, staff, and students during this time. School nurses understand and are prepared for emergencies, crises, and outbreaks that may occur in the school setting. Every day we collect data, assess, evaluate, plan, and implement for the well-being of the students and staff in our schools.

There is no doubt that this is just the beginning of more outbreaks from swine flu in our schools. As a school nurse, I know my job in the schools will continue to be educating students and staff about the virus, preparing for outbreaks, and collecting information to use as a tool in the crisis prevention and intervention phases. As more complex health issues arise in our school settings, the importance and necessity of school nurses will only increase. As advocates for students, we must also be advocates for nurses in the school setting.

Beth H. Wipf, BSN, RN
Florida

Multitasking

Being responsible for numerous schools containing populations of medically fragile children mixed in with the regular school population is a challenge; therefore, school nurses need to know when to: delegate minor incidents, take care of emergencies, supervise, perform health care assessments, educate teachers, involve community services, and counsel those in immediate need of assistance. Examine for yourself the stories of how school nurses are the master "multidoers" in today's age of modern technology.

Perfecting the Art of Multitasking

I am one of five, full-time, credentialed school nurses that serve a population of about thirteen thousand five hundred students (K-12, including special and alternative education).

For the most part, parity of numbers served by the school nurse is about equal. My four other colleagues each have about three thousand students that they serve. I have between twelve hundred and fourteen hundred students because I cover special education three days per week, alternative education one day per week, and one elementary school.

When I look back, I realize how much has changed in such a short period of time. Eight years ago, when I started my career as a special education school nurse, I covered anywhere from one hundred to two hundred fifty students with special needs. That was close to the National Association of School Nurses' (NASN) recommended ratio for working with severely handicapped special needs students, which is one nurse for every one hundred twenty-five students. For students in the general population, the NASN recommends one school nurse for every seven hundred fifty well students.

Since that time, many things have drastically changed in our student population. Some of the most pronounced changes that we have seen are in the area of the advanced technological needs that our students require. We now have students who are dependent on ventilators and gastrostomy, cecostomy, and jejunostomy tubes. Years ago, many of these students might have been in specialty care centers, schools for the deaf or the blind, or children's rehab centers because of their disabilities.

I oversee students with chronic and life-threatening health conditions, including diabetes, asthma, food allergies, cerebral palsy, spina bifida, epilepsy, Rett Syndrome, autism, heart conditions, and so on. On a typical day, I will assist students at four to six different school sites to perform procedures (gastrostomy tube feedings, diabetes management, bladder catheterizations, etc.), screen vision and hearing or scoliosis, and educate staff on the use of Epi-Pens®, rectal Diastat®, or Glucagon, or put up a bulletin board on health promotion outside one of the many health offices I work in.

The daily workload for school nurses has kept pace with the increased dependency on technology. Because of this technology, we have user-friendly equipment that allows children to attend their community schools with the aid of advanced nursing requirements. On an average day, it is not unusual to find us doing bladder catheterizations, tube feedings, and insulin pump monitoring (not to mention the daily monitoring of multiple blood sugars testing) to approximately fifty identified Type I diabetic students.

The daily requirements of credentialed school nurses for maintaining the health of fragile populations, combined with mandated assessments, has clearly changed the typical school nurse's day. This is why it is imperative to have qualified licensed and credentialed school nurses. Schools need someone who can see the difference between a harmless bump on the head and a concussion, someone who can educate teachers and other staff members how to recognize a student with diabetes experiencing a low blood sugar count before the student passes out and slips into a coma.

As a school nurse, I find myself constantly growing and learning. I love working with the diverse populations. In the past, I have worked as a certified oncology nurse, in home health as a case manager, in various departments throughout local hospitals, including rehabilitation and behavioral health, and as a case manager for group homes for adults with disabilities. My current job as a school nurse can be very demanding sometimes and multifaceted at all times, and I constantly strive to perfect the art of multitasking. Most of all, my job is the most rewarding job I have ever done! I love that no two days are ever the same.

Julie Parker, RN
California

JUST IN TIME

Quality school nursing requires additional skills and knowledge that are unique to the school setting. These skills and knowledge are not otherwise developed in the traditional health care system. Similarities do exist with these three basic perspectives of prevention, management, and intervention.

Prevention is the goal for healthy students to become healthy adults. Prevention education works to support positive student and staff health through the use of recognition and early intervention, as well as healthy lifestyle choices.

Management requires the school nurse to provide and develop an effective health care plan for chronic diseases. The school health care plan serves to prevent negative outcomes from a disease by prompting teachers and administrators to recognize early signs and symptoms and to take action, which includes notifying the school nurse and (when the situation requires it) deploying emergency responders.

Intervention is accomplished by prompt delivery of safe, effective nursing care and medical treatments or procedures. Quality intervention equal to that expected in the health care system is mandatory. Without provision of quality care from licensed professionals, harm or death may result.

Schools hold large and diverse age groups and populations for eight to ten hours per day. The schools could possibly house the largest range of health issues and unknown health problems when compared to any other workplace or educational setting. The needs represented in a daily school routine are of great interest to us. We would like to work more closely with the physicians serving these populations and be prepared to respond with quality outcomes. We see ourselves as extensions of the physicians' practices, and we are often underutilized.

Prior to the nursing requirements for schools, teachers and teaching assistants were left to meet the increasing teaching demands placed on them as well as deal with many health issues in the growing student population. Teachers are both relieved and grateful for the support the school nurse provides in keeping our students healthy and symptom free.

A female student in our ninth grade was struggling with academic expectations. Not feeling very well for days upon end only added to her challenge. She was from a family with a stepfather and stepsiblings. The mother and student had had rounds of arguments through the years pertaining to grades, boys, attitudes, and expectations.

The young girl visited the school nurse's office only twice in that particular school year and had never been considered a frequent visitor. She had vague complaints that were inconsistent with any specific disease process. A gut feeling led the school nurse to determine that her complaints were valid enough to warrant an examination, but she was not able to put together the pieces without a basic laboratory analysis. The teacher, counselor, and school nurse had a parent conference just prior to Thanksgiving. The school nurse needs to be part of the child study team and be considered as the medical expert for the school setting, since most school districts do not employ physicians.

The school nurse urged the mother and student to seek a medical examination for her complaints, including the need for updated immunizations.

Later that afternoon, the student collapsed. She was rushed to the local emergency room, where she was found to have a blood glucose level of over eight hundred. The student was admitted, treated, and returned to school to report that she had insulin-dependent diabetes.

Although the school nurse does not have the luxury of prompt medical laboratory testing available in the school health office, she does have knowledge and a familiarity of people on the verge of a health crisis. How many more situations are out there waiting to be identified? Students and staff alike are in need of the skills and knowledge provided by a qualified school nurse.

Melanie Sharpton, RN
Alabama

Phone Calls to E-mail

There was a time when I made phone calls to correspond with parents, administrators, doctors, local school nurses, and other community personnel for medical and administrative decisions.

With the introduction of new-age technology, I rarely communicate with other human beings via the telephone anymore. I do not even have to get off my chair to speak to anyone; I just e-mail! A considerable amount of my day is spent either sending or reading e-mails.

Each day begins with me sitting in front of my computer sending e-mails to the principal and staff to learn what happened the night before, including any non-emergencies in school that need my attention. Once that is done, I start the task of e-mailing conference calls to medical doctors, local community administrators, and in-district school nurses. I respond to e-mail questions and concerns that parents have about in-school illnesses, and include questions that I have regarding handwritten notes that their physicians scan and e-mail to me.

Many school districts now have student health cards computerized, but this doubles the workload for those school nurses that still keep hardcopies of student health forms on file. Of course, computerized health cards do keep student information consolidated, but not to the point yet of effectively streamlining the administrative side of school nursing.

I love my students and their families, the personal contact that I have with school personnel, and my job. I will gracefully accept the new-age technology and e-mail to "one and all."

And of course, I still get the occasional joke on my e-mail!

Janne M. DeMarco, MS, BS, RN, LPN, CSN
New Jersey

Who Am I and What Hat Should I Wear Today?

My job description as a school nurse:

> *Baccalaureate needed, with at least five years' experience in public health and emergency nursing. Must work thirty hours a week. Must be able to provide health direction for students and staff of approximately twelve hundred, as well as review and write procedures and protocols. Candidate must demonstrate ability to interface with and give direction to parents.*

This is my job, and I love it! When I answered the newspaper ad approximately twenty years ago, I had no idea what doors it would open for me. I thought my expertise in emergency nursing would be what I would bring to this job, but I couldn't have been more wrong. I thought it might be a little boring, but I would find ways around that by being innovative and teaching kids to learn to care for themselves. I would also teach parents to better care for their children and teach staff about preventive care and how to access the care they need. I wrote grants and was the Title IX coordinator, a member of the safety committee, a department of transportation representative, the wellness coordinator, and a member of numerous other committees. These responsibilities somehow turned a thirty-hour week into a fifty-hour week, which was not part of the plan but part of the job.

Writing health care plans (IHP) for students with medical and psychological needs was an important aspect, but certainly not the most important part of my job. Providing emergency care when needed was also important. However, the privilege of being part of numerous staff efforts and special projects with students throughout the years has been the job's hallmark. This job has made me happy and made me sad, it has made me humble and reduced me to tears of sympathy, but mostly it has made me grateful that I could share my skills with so many people.

It isn't a job of putting Band-Aids on kids, but sometimes it's putting Band-Aids on their hearts. It's a job of showing teens the right road to travel and of being a role model for all. It is not a road traveled by many, but I have been privileged to follow it and it has become my passion!

Marcia Howard, BSN, RN, PHN
Montana

Intervention

Teaching a child how to take care of their personal hygiene is intervention. Recommending community services to a family in need is intervention. Working with other school nurses in the community to eradicate a disease is intervention. Sending home a sick child is intervention. The list is endless regarding how often a school nurse uses intervention in caring for students. Gain insight and knowledge regarding school health services by reading how the school nurse reaches out through "intervention."

SUBSTITUTE MOM

I have been a school nurse for nineteen years. Prior to my time as a school nurse, I was a supervisor to staff nurses in a thirty-two bed, full-service hospital in a small town. I was an office nurse to a family physician for thirteen years. I appreciated on a daily basis the knowledge and expertise I gained at an excellent three-year hospital school of nursing. My health education skills were honed when I obtained my degree in health studies at Western Michigan University.

I have seen as many as 19,600 students a year, but average about sixteen thousand. I see between one hundred and one hundred thirty students a day (not counting staff, parents, and community members who come in or call my clinic). Of those, fifty to seventy-five are sick and injured students. The remainder of those seen in a day are the routine head checks. I am the only nurse for 1,475 culturally diverse students in grades preschool through twelve.

With these numbers, I rarely get coffee or lunch breaks. These are usually taken as I see and treat. Lunch recess times are my busiest. Besides treating the usual bumps and scrapes of recess, I have had a possible fractured ankle, possible concussion, and soiled pants to deal with all at the same time. It is all about prioritizing, triaging, and multitasking.

Besides the emergency or urgent issues, I care for students with chronic conditions, such as congenital anomalies, joint pain, asthma, heart conditions, hypertension, and diabetes. Diabetes seems to be more prevalent now than ever before. In my tenure, I started out with none to one or two diabetic students just seven years ago. Now I have seven diabetic students in my school district. Three of those students handle their own care, while the other four require my hands-on expertise. Four of these students became diabetic at an early age (five to seven years old), which seems to be the norm for diabetic children.

I also deal with diabetes in a different form. Type II has been occurring in my overweight and obese teenagers. They were usually children who disliked exercise or physical education. If they did participate, it was at about half the speed, and they would get exhausted. These are the children who were allowed constant indoor video-game activity. I feel for these students, who missed out on the physical rush you get from the camaraderie of outdoor activity.

Trying to maintain healthy basic nutrition for our students is a huge challenge for our food service department. There are issues of budget constraints, finicky eaters, people pleasing, and the challenge of making healthy foods look and taste appetizing. Because dietary habits start at home, picky eating habits spill over to school. It's all well and good to have children eat more fruits, vegetables, and whole grains at school, but this is many times not even ventured at home. I can't bear to go to the cafeteria and see all the delicious, healthy, nutritious food thrown away! We try to teach these children about nutrition and the food pyramid, but such healthy habits have to start at home so that a basis is set before starting school.

We work hard in school through curriculums, discussion groups, health fairs, and role modeling so that young people are educated on the health and legal issues involved. As school nurses and educators, all we can do is just get the correct information out to the children and pray they use it to make informed decisions.

My fellow staff members have to continue to remind me how hard we try to inform and that we can't always be there for our students. "Marilyn, you can't be with them 24/7." But there are numerous times I wish I was there for those students who have to get themselves up and off to school by themselves. These kids sometimes just catch the bus, halfway dressed with one piece of pajamas still on, and have had no breakfast and no one to hug or kiss them good-bye as they fly out the door.

In my first few years as a school nurse, I had a first-grade student who would come and hug me as soon as she entered the school and the last thing before she got on the bus. I finally mentioned this to her older half-sister. She informed me that her mother worked long hours every day. We had a motivational speaker at our school that year for our first staff in-service of the year. He informed us that it was okay to tell these children we loved them. So almost that whole school year, I eagerly welcomed or said good-bye, hugged, and told this student I loved her. As the school year came toward the end, the times she came into the clinic became fewer and further between. I realized I had hopefully filled her emotional need at that time in her life.

There have, however, been instances in my school nursing career that hugs and "I love you's" aren't enough. To see children physically and mentally abused, neglected, unloved, and at the brunt of a relative's anger tears my heart out. Thank goodness I have supportive staff, administration, and outside resources to rely on in these circumstances. I am lucky to have social workers and counselors on our staff from whom I can seek advice. I have a good working relationship with our county social services department, which I never hesitate to call on. If I feel that the need is dire, I will continue to contact and pursue their office until I get their full attention.

There is one point I must touch on in this discussion of school nursing. I would never consider working one minute of my job without having full coverage nursing liability of my own. Yes, you are covered under the Good

Samaritan laws and by your school district, but never go without having some protection of your own. You cannot function as a nurse anytime in your life without liability insurance. School nurses are many times the only nurses in their district, diagnosing and functioning as a registered professional nurse. We stick ourselves out there, exposing ourselves to the chance of litigation every minute of the day. So this is my advice to every registered professional nurse out there on the school's front lines: get liability insurance to cover yourself immediately.

About ten years ago, I was asked if I would mentor college nursing students. At first, I was intimidated at the thought. What could they learn from me? But in my crazy, hectic schedule, I realized what an asset they could be to me. As I started to work with them, I found myself sharing my work experiences and nursing expertise with evolving student nurses. They could subsequently gain health, medical, and nursing experience, knowledge as well as academic credit. In the last ten years, I have watched these students grow in their nursing skills and knowledge, people skills, and managerial experience, as well as mature in life. I feel I have in many ways helped my nursing profession stem nursing shortages by adding these many wonderful, excited, experienced nurses into the field. I feel this is one of the biggest contributions to my nursing legacy.

Marilyn L. Hebert, BS, RN
Michigan

School Nurses Are Public Health Allies

There is a proven successful way to address the pressing health needs of today's youth—one that is cost effective and readily able to be implemented, but unfortunately often overlooked and taken for granted.

This program reaches across all cultural and linguistic groups and includes athletes and those with disabilities, leaving no child behind. It addresses childhood weight and obesity issues, as well as eating disorders and general health education about good nutrition.

For those with dental disease, incomplete immunizations, or vision or hearing deficits, this program goes looking for previously undetected problems and promptly responds to the need for care. It implements prevention programs to encourage healthy choices and deals with issues of substance abuse, including illegal drugs, alcohol, and tobacco use.

It teaches about physical development, personal hygiene, puberty, and maturation, and intervenes to deal with STDs, pregnancy, and teenage parenthood. It helps young people work out relational issues and gender identity questions. Where there is homelessness, truancy, violence, or mental health concerns, such as depression or suicidal feelings, it intercedes. When a child has a long-term health condition, such as diabetes, asthma, ADD/ADHD, life-threatening allergies, or HIV/AIDS, the providers of this program are there for the day-to-day monitoring, care, and intervention.

For the looming communicable illnesses of TB or MRSA, the annoyance of lice, or the remote possibility of bird flu or smallpox, these individuals are on the front line of surveillance and are there in the event of a mass casualty. They provide first aid and emergency care on a daily basis, connect families to primary care providers, and facilitate the enrollment of children in state health insurance programs. When a child develops symptoms of acute illness, these health care providers perform assessment and intervention and implement a plan of care that often keeps a mildly ill child functioning so that a parent can remain in the workplace.

The program that delivers these services (and more) is well-known but not well understood or recognized for its value. The providers of this health care initiative are most often appreciated but paid less than colleagues with similar education levels in parallel roles. This program supports the efforts of local public health departments, reduces emergency room visits, keeps health insurance costs down, and contributes to the general welfare of every community. *This program is school health services, as provided by school nurses.*

Every child deserves to have access to a school nurse in ratios that meet the standard guidelines of one school nurse for every seven hundred fifty well students. School nurses support academic success by ensuring that children are healthy and ready to learn. The greatest teaching on earth will not be effective unless a child is physically and emotionally receptive.

For the sake of our students and in support of the educational process, promote strong school health service programs, pay a school nurse a salary at least comparable to a teacher, and thank a school nurse today.

Wendy Doremus, MS, RN, NP-BC
Massachusetts

Ponytail Lesson

I became a school health aide thirteen years ago, after my last child entered preschool. Previously, I had spent the time at home, taking care of my family. It had been ten years since I was part of the workforce.

I had not wanted to be a part of nursing in any capacity, but without a degree and needing more skills, school health seemed a reasonable place to start. I went through all the required steps and was very fortunate to become a part of my current school family. As I've told anyone who cared to listen, your work environment makes all the difference. It has to be more than just a workplace, more than just a job. Substituting at other schools has given me a good concept of other work environments and a great appreciation for mine. Through experience, I can safely say that the staff (family) I work with is the absolute best. We have differences, but we work together very well. I enjoy going to work every day.

Children are the most fun people in the world. The stories that they share make you laugh, and sometimes they make you sad. For them, life is about the families that love them, their friends, the fun they have at home and school. They ask so many questions; they want to know everything. Sometimes it reminds you of how we take so many things for granted in our lives.

Besides the daily care of scrapes, bumps, bruises, and occasional nosebleeds, there's always a time to make an actual difference in a child's life. We have our share of families who are large and struggle to make ends meet. Many times a child will be unnoticed. He or she will wear the same clothes for days. The hair is unkempt. Self-esteem is nearly nonexistent. I had one such child that sticks in my memory.

Her clothes were usually too big, hand-me-downs from older siblings. Her hair was sticky, tangled, and long, and it appeared unclean. She would come to the health room with a stomachache. After some rest, she would return to the classroom. We spoke of family. As she was the youngest in her family coming through my school, I was already familiar with several of her older sisters. She hid behind her hair and spoke softly.

One day I asked her about brushing her hair. She had many excuses: "I don't have my own brush" and "I don't know how." I went on to advise her about the importance of appearance. I stressed how pretty she would look if she brushed her hair every morning and tied it back. In this way, everyone would be able to see her pretty smile and her pretty face. She could come to me in the morning, and I could help her to do her hair.

In the weeks that followed, I started to see a change in her. It started with her hair. It appeared cleaner. She had it brushed and pulled back into a ponytail. I would watch for her, just to see that she continued the grooming. I was not disappointed. Her clothes started to fit better, and they were cleaner as well. She wasn't running around with shoes that were too big, and she was no longer barefoot.

It was a wonderful feeling. I was able to watch this child bloom. She no longer came to the health room with stomachaches. The only time I ever saw her was when she was on campus going to class with friends.

Of all the injuries and illnesses that I've taken care of, no memory could top this one for me. It is my foremost memory of how I can really care for a child. I can make a difference in a child's life, other than taking a temperature or putting on a bandage. I've had a few other cases similar to this one, and each one touches me in the same way.

Phyllis E. Kobayashi, School Health Aide
Hawaii

Together We Can Make a
Difference to a Child

Working in the largest elementary school in an urban, disadvantaged district with over twelve hundred students and two hundred staff is a challenging experience. This school is allotted at least two certified school nurses, and previously we had two full-time nurses and a half-time nurse. This year, I am the only full-time nurse in this school. There are a myriad of challenges, and there are no two days alike. Every day in the school presents a new story.

As the medical person in the building, I wear a lot of hats. I also sit on the school's intervention and referral services team. We had a second grader with learning and emotional issues. The aunt now has legal custody of the child. The team recommended that the legal guardian, as soon as possible, take this child for a medical work-up in the local hospital.

As the school nurse, I wrote a letter to the chief of the pediatric clinic; a week later, I received a phone call from the doctor in the hospital, who stated that the hospital wanted to help this child as much as the school did.

This is a perfect picture of a great collaboration within the community, when the school, hospital, and home get together to help a child succeed academically as well as develop a sound mind and body.

Rosamarie Cruz, MEd, BSN, RN, CSN
New Jersey

From Head Lice to Budget Cuts

During the second month of my school nursing career, a mother called to say that she found a small brown bug in her daughter's hair and could I please examine her daughter's hair. I called the nurse at another school in our town to help me, as I never had seen pediculosis (head lice) in all my years as a hospital nurse or corporate nurse. The other school nurse came to my school and taught me how and what to look for in examining for head lice. Consequently, a number of students were found to have head lice, and notes were sent home to parents. Other schools in the district were having the same problem.

From October to November of that year, I spent hours checking schoolchildren's heads. I thought at the time, if this is what school nursing is all about, then I'm going to quit! Thank goodness the town school nurses and I were able to get the outbreak of lice under control. During the summer months, there is the problem of an infestation due to children attending camps or playing games that require close contact that spreads the lice. It became policy to check all children in the elementary schools on the second day of return to school in September to avert any outbreaks.

During the next few years, many of the elementary school nurses had to service two schools. This policy at times made it difficult to provide full-time health care to the students. At a later date, when each elementary school had a full-time nurse, teaching health education courses in family life became part of the nurses' daily responsibility. If there were an emergency, the classroom teacher would take over the class while the nurse tended to the emergency. Teaching is enjoyable, and I felt the students were interested in learning about health. The difficulty was trying to include the teaching while fulfilling all the other duties that were required of the school nurse.

Within the school district, necessary budget cuts affected special education students being sent out of district to private schools. To remedy this situation, it became the norm to mainstream medically fragile children into the general classroom. Thus, the responsibility of special medical attention to these students fell to the already overscheduled school nurse. Most of the school days are filled with good times, but the reality of having medically fragile children in school brings into focus the sad times when children may succumb to an illness and can no longer live a full and happy life. The sadness has an effect on everyone at the school, including the entire staff and the students' classmates.

I have enjoyed my work as a school nurse each and every day for the past twenty-five years. Obviously, I never did quit! I have met and cared for many students during those years and will truly miss the rapport that I shared with them.

Mary A. O'Neill, MA, RN, CSN
New Jersey

It's the Little Things That Count

I have experienced the joy of teaching kindergarteners how to wash their hands via a video called *Scrubby Bear*. When they see me come down the hallway, they chant, "Hi, you are Scrubby Bear! Don't get sick. Wash up quick." I have taught nutrition, safety, body changes, drugs, tobacco, and blood-borne pathogens. I have had parents tell me they were impressed by the health information their children have discussed, and students say health class was the best part of their day. Of course, I wish there were staying power in the lessons and that all students would continue to use what they learned, but I am realistic and hope that a few will follow through and others may get it the next time around.

I have helped numerous students get dental, vision, and medical care that they otherwise could not afford. I have lobbied for students' health needs. There was a student who was having daily headaches, who needed money to pay for six root canals. I was able to find a private donor willing to look at the child's needs. Sure, these things are little things, not something you would hear about in the news. Some students' parents teach healthy habits and care for their children's health. But for those students who do not have such parents, having a school nurse as a health advocate does make a difference.

I have cared for students with medications, fractures, concussions, infections, diabetes, allergies, asthma, communicable diseases, and more. I have ridden with students to the ER. I have been the "go to" person for body hygiene or inappropriate touching issues. Yet, I find that many see nurses as those who "take care of students' boo-boos," which were the words used by my principal before the school board when I was awarded tenure. Just this past year, a retiring nurse was almost not replaced because the administration was considering hiring unlicensed aides to cover the nurse's office. I was told that it was just to take care of the boo-boos. The question I asked was, "Who decides if it is just a boo-boo?"

What about the second grader who fell in gym and knocked out a permanent tooth? I had a staff member bring the tooth to my office, and I put it in milk and called the parents and the dentist. The child has a healthy tooth today because I was in the building. That is what makes my job as a school nurse worthwhile, one day at a time, one student at a time. It's the little things that count.

Sharon L. King, RN, NCSN
Wyoming

First Year

Wow, what a year! When I took on the job as a school nurse this year, I thought it would be a good way to ease into working. I had just graduated from nursing school in June 2007. Nine months later, I am now sure it was not the ease into nursing I thought it was going to be, but I love every minute of my job.

Being a first-year nurse, as well as a first-year school nurse, is an exciting challenge and a big responsibility. I am currently the nurse for two different districts, totaling five schools that have sixteen hundred kids in all. It is up to me to know if any of these kids have health concerns and are not up–to-date on their immunizations. It is my job to assess and take care of them in the event of illness or injury. I also have to train the staff so that, if necessary, they can care for these kids in my absence. From concussions to broken bones, asthma attacks to allergies, bee stings to head lice, vision and scoliosis screening to AIDS/HIV talks, it is all up to me.

There are some days that could be classified as light or easy, such as when the day adds up to just handing out Band-Aids, ice packs, and a few kind words. To me those interactions with the kids are just as important as the days spent on my feet with a line of sick children. Whether it is helping them figure out why they are in trouble or helping them decide what they want to do with their lives, you get attached to these kids. You want them to succeed, and you truly get affected by what some of them have to go home to.

This year has made me realize how much I love being a nurse and how being a school nurse is just as important to the community as being a nurse in a hospital. I am very blessed to have the opportunity to be a part of kids' lives and wouldn't trade the experience for anything.

Domichellei Walker, RN
Washington

Lessons Learned

Originally, I heard through all of my hospital nursing friends that school nursing was an easy job, a cakewalk compared to the demanding, difficult work at the hospital. Since I have become a school nurse, my perception has changed greatly. School nursing is a lot of things, but easy is not one of them.

When I did my internship with a certified school nurse, I had my eyes opened to the reality of school nursing. I found out that most school nurses have more than one school and they may not be very close together, requiring you to get into your car to drive to the other school. My cooperating school nurse taught me calmness, kindness, and patience when trying to deal with an emergency over the phone while driving. I found out that the school nurse not only takes care of the students and staff, but also the parents of the students and sometimes the relatives of staff. I realized the specific knowledge that a school nurse must have concerning rules and regulations. I saw that a nurse is the minority, as compared to the hospital, where nurses are the majority.

The amount of autonomy, independence, and self-sufficiency that a school nurse needs is vast. I learned that the school secretary can be your best friend, because she knows most of the children and their parents. I found teachers to be extremely pleasant to work with and was surprised to see how much they valued the school nurse's opinion. I discovered the joy that comes from working with children of all ages. I absolutely love to see their smiles after witnessing their tears. There is no better feeling than to have a first grader draw you a picture and proudly give it to you the day after you had taken care of their scraped knee.

It took a year after I got my school nurse certification to finally get a job. Luckily, I work in a school district with another nurse, who is one of the sweetest and most giving people I've ever met. I have two schools. I work with preschool children and with middle school students. I love both ages, even though they are completely different. Hearing three- and four-year-olds sing happy songs every morning is the best way ever to start out a workday. Making a long-lasting bond with a middle school student who feels that they just can't talk to anyone else about their problems is extremely gratifying. These days the cabinets at both of my schools are covered with students' drawings, a reminder of how rewarding being a school nurse can be.

Robin Halemeyer, BSN, RN, CSN
Illinois

A Piece of My Heart

Rising from my chair, I gently closed my office door and switched off the light. Returning to my seat, I sat down and fully exhaled. Then the tears came. My morning had been spent interviewing and obtaining medical histories from pregnant teenage girls. There was nothing unusual about this activity. Many times each week, I performed these tasks as part of my job as a school nurse in an alternative school for pregnant and parenting teenage girls. Over the years, I have heard many sad stories from my students, but this particular morning the stories seemed sadder than usual and I felt I was losing a piece of my heart. The last student I interviewed was "Susie," and her story beat them all.

Susie was fifteen when her boyfriend left her after hearing of her pregnancy. She also had medical issues as well as family issues. After hearing her story, I hardly knew where to start with the interventions. Obviously, Susie needed to receive medical care as soon as possible. She needed to speak with a social worker and a counselor about the services they offered, and she needed to be referred for further counseling pertaining to the possibility of adoption or parenting classes.

Susie attended our school during her pregnancy. After delivering her baby, she decided to keep it. But there was another twist to the story. Her baby was born with several lifelong medical problems.

In spite of all the obstacles Susie had faced in her short life, she embraced motherhood like a duck takes to water. Although the baby had medical problems, she made the decision to keep it and, as she said, "to give it the love I never had as a child." She blossomed under the care of her foster parents. Susie went back to her home campus when the baby was several months old, and I was unable to follow up on her after that.

Some would say that Susie should not have kept the baby—that she would fail as a parent because of her past. What I witnessed in Susie was the resiliency of the human spirit. She was a survivor. Even though life had beaten her down, Susie never gave up. She looked forward to the opportunity she had to accelerate her education at our school. She wanted to be an example to her younger siblings.

I was very proud and honored to have helped Susie find her way to becoming a responsible young parent by having her participate in child development and parenting classes, by assisting her to find prenatal care, by following up with her to make sure she was keeping her prenatal appointments, and by encouraging her to finish her high school education.

The morning that I interviewed her, I closed my door and shed private tears. This I did because all I could see was failure in her future. I felt Susie had too many obstacles to overcome. She proved me wrong, and I am glad she did. When sad stories pour in, students like Susie are what keep me going. When I start doubting if a student can make it through the mire of life, I think of Susie, and hope enters the picture again.

During my fourteen years as a school nurse, I have worked with all levels of students, from newborns to high school. I have worked alone, with no clerical help or health aide, in an elementary school with a population of over twelve hundred students. That situation was my baptism by fire into the world of school nursing. At the time, the school district in which I worked had no formal support for new school nurses. You either sank or swam. Today there is a much better system in place to help new nurses adjust to their roles. Now, there is at least one registered nurse on each of the fifty-two campuses in our district. I took the advice of my first nursing supervisor, who said, "School nursing is what you make of it." I also adhered to the advice of a nursing colleague: "Bloom where you are planted."

To be honest, I went into school nursing because I wanted a change from the hectic pace of the hospital OB-GYN floor, where I would have to work every other weekend, never being able to take a vacation around the holidays. I also had three small children and wanted to spend time with my family. After working alone at my elementary school, I began to like the autonomy that this position offered me. It forced me to trust my own decisions and to be creative with my problem-solving skills. I found I also enjoyed teaching different health topics and hosting different health presentations with community resources. Developing relationships with "frequent-flier" students was challenging, but interesting.

It took me about three years to find my niche in school nursing. That niche came when I took the position I now have at the teen parenting campus. When I first came here, there was also a large unit of severe and profoundly handicapped students. Thus, my clinical skills became very important since these students had many medications and treatments and were very fragile. It was fun and rewarding to get to know these students, with their individual personalities.

Because of my clinical background in obstetrics, I truly love working with pregnant teenage girls. They can be very challenging, but I feel I do make a difference in many lives. Some of these young women see me as a teacher, some see me as a counselor, and some view me as a foster mom. I have a passion for encouraging these young women to become responsible citizens, good moms, and high school graduates, with hopes for postsecondary schooling. There is also an in-house day care at our facility, and I enjoy seeing the babies every day. It takes much patience to instill adequate parenting skills in teen moms. There are a range of issues, including correct administration of medications to babies, how to prevent illness and diaper rash, hygiene concerns, how and what to feed babies at different stages, and safety issues, such as using car seats.

The biggest reward for me is seeing these girls, who came to my school lacking self-esteem and with low motivation, graduate and walk out the door confident in themselves and their parenting abilities. Because of the assistance they received, they are able to conquer their worlds, and for that they can have a piece of my heart.

Vici McClure, BSN, RN
Texas

THE EIGHTH-GRADE GRADUATION

What an exciting time of the year at the middle school! It was the end of May, and the school year was almost done and all of the students and staff were getting restless and ready for summer vacation. When I became a school nurse, I thought my job would be taking care of students with injuries and illnesses and the accompanying paperwork. I was so wrong. A school nurse is also part parent, part teacher, part social worker, part guidance counselor, and any other thing that comes up in the day-to-day world of children.

As the school nurse, I had developed some great relationships with so many of the students in the eighth grade, and I knew I would miss them greatly when they moved on to high school next year. Several students had asked me if I was going to attend their eighth-grade graduation ceremony. It was only my second year at the school and I hadn't gone to it the previous year, so I hadn't really considered it. But once students started asking me to go, I decided that I should go to send them off. I talked to my principal about it, and he told me the school nurse doesn't usually go but I was more than welcome—as a matter of fact, they needed someone to help pin on the flower corsages that were ordered for the occasion. I was so excited. The eighth graders were feeling so special and really looking forward to the ceremony.

About four days before the graduation was scheduled, at the end of the school day on a Friday, one of the eighth-grade teachers, Mrs. Green, came to see me and told me that two of her male students, Mike and Rich, didn't have dress shoes for the occasion and couldn't afford to buy them. She had already located dress clothes for them. She wanted to know if there was a fund we could use to buy them shoes. We had a nurse's fund, but it was typically used for eyeglasses, physical exam fees, and other health-related needs of the students. I called our school social worker to see if he had any dress shoes lying around, and he said he didn't. I thought of our superintendent and called him. He asked why I didn't just buy new shoes for both of them. I explained to him that several employees, including the district's bookkeeper and some teachers, had already offered to buy new shoes, and we were trying to avoid having any one person have to buy new shoes. So we left it at that and went home for the weekend.

I woke up really early on Saturday morning and decided to go to a few yard sales, as I did many Saturday mornings. At the very first sale I went to, I found two pairs of men's brand-new leather dress shoes that a man had bought and they ended up not fitting him. I was ecstatic and went home to call Mrs. Green and let her know that the problem was solved that easily; we had two pairs of shoes in brand-new condition that would be perfect for the graduation ceremony.

I came in really excited on Monday morning and found that the social worker had brought in a perfect pair of shoes and the superintendent had also brought in shoes. I was ecstatic. The school was overflowing with people who really cared about the students and went to the trouble to find shoes. It may seem like a trivial thing, but to students who can't afford them, it is a big deal. I put the extra shoes away for next year because I knew someone else would need them.

Mrs. Green sent the two students in to try on the shoes, and they each chose the pair that they liked and that fit perfectly. Mike smiled shyly and asked if he got to keep the shoes because he would like to wear them to church. He said he had been wearing his old worn-out sneakers to church but always tried to hide them because he was embarrassed about them. I told him, "Of course, you can keep them; they are yours now." Rich put his shoes on and started strutting around my office and liked them so much that he decided to wear them all day at school that day with his blue jeans.

I attended the eighth-grade graduation that year and was beaming with pride, as if they were my own children graduating. I helped pin on corsages, listened to their nervous giggles, and helped to get everyone lined up. I got several hugs, smiles, and waves from students and their parents; I felt as though they appreciated me being there to share in their celebration. I even had a few tears in my eyes thinking of how I would miss these kids I had spent so much time with, but I knew they had to move on and continue with their education. Growth and transitions are an important part of life.

I'll never forget how such a small thing made the students so happy and made me feel so good inside, knowing how much those I work with care about the students. I'm glad I went to the graduation ceremony and plan to attend every year. A school nurse wears many hats, not just a nursing cap, and the feeling is wonderful.

Robin Halemeyer, BSN, RN, CSN
Illinois

The Blue Denim Hat

Although the events in this story happened about twenty years ago, it is a story that will be forever with me.

It was a rainy Friday morning when a student I will call Jane came into the school nurse's office. She had asthma, and I thought the weather might be affecting her; instinctively, I got out my stethoscope and bent over to check her breathing. She wasn't wheezing—she was crying. I couldn't tell which was coming down harder, the rain or the tears.

Jane's parents separated when she was four, and she lived with her father until she was thirteen. Jane decided at thirteen years old to live on the streets. Life on the streets is hard. Jane had to make tough decisions as to how she was going to survive living on the streets and not end up a "statistic." Now, she was living with her aunt.

I sat there with her for a while, knowing there were more tears to come. Finally, she looked up and said, "You remember my friend, Sarah? She was shot and killed in a drive-by shooting last night." Jane reached out, and I hugged her and let her continue. She explained that her friend would be buried in a pine box tomorrow, with no one at her funeral. She told me no one gave a damn about her when she was alive and no one would give a damn about her now that she was dead. I tried to console her by asking about Sarah's family. Jane just shook her head and told me that Sarah had not lived with her parents since she was ten years old. There was nothing I could say to change any of this, so I just sat with her.

Then, with the wisdom of a troubled sixteen-year-old, Jane said something I will never forget. She stood up, walked to the door, turned, and looked me straight in the eye as she said, "You know something, Mrs. K.? Life isn't fair, and this isn't supposed to happen. Moms are supposed to buy blue denim hats for their little girls and take them to the park to swing."

I thought about Jane and her friend Sarah as I locked my office that day. The rain had cleared, so on my way home, I stopped at Wal-Mart and bought my own daughter a blue denim hat. I picked my daughter up from day care, put that hat on her head, and took her to the park to swing. For the longest time, I stood there and watched that little girl and the rhythm of her and the swing.

My daughter is in college now, but her blue denim hat still hangs on her bedpost. I think about Jane and wonder whatever happened to her. She was right. Life isn't fair. But my life is richer now because of her.

Jean Anne Kamrath, MSFL, BSN, RN
Nebraska

Contributors

Anne E. Allen, BSN, RN, OCN, obtained her bachelor's of science degree from Montana State University and is certified as an oncology nurse. She and her husband, Wailes, live and work on the family ranch with their young daughters, Addison and Aubrey. When the little ones are napping and Anne is off duty, she enjoys crafts, quilting, and scrapbooking.

Patricia H. Allocca, LCSW, RN, CSN, received an associate's degree in nursing from County College of Morris and Caldwell College in New Jersey. Broadening her skills, she obtained a master's degree in social work from New York University and works as a licensed clinical social worker in her own private practice. Patricia is a single mother of two energetic boys, Christopher and Nicholas. Together they enjoy skiing, snowboarding, and skateboarding.

Eunice Arendt, RN, a veteran nurse for over thirty-two years, has been married to her husband, Tim, for nearly that long. They share three daughters and seven grandchildren. Eunice is co-owner of a motorcycle accessories business and enjoys the stress relief of motorcycle travel.

Amy Jayne Barnes, MA, BSN, RN, a School Nurse from 1994-1995, then again in 1997 to the present time for the Lee County School District in Fort Myers, Florida. Amy earned both her bachelor's and her master's degree from the University of South Florida. In 2003, Amy was published in the book *A Long Way from Henry Street: A Collection of Stories from School Nurses.* Amy has been recognized for her professionalism in many circles.

Linda Betley, MSN, RN, is now working on her dream of becoming a nursing instructor. She earned her bachelor's degree from the University of Massachusetts and her master's degree from the University of Hartford, Connecticut. Her husband, Robert, and she have been married for over twenty-six years and have three grown children. Linda has discovered the Syracuse Opera and a local jazz club and symphony.

Wanda Bouvier, RNC, has worked in maternity nursing, the emergency room, a medical center, and most recently, as a school nurse in a high school. She earned her associate's degree in science and nursing at Castleton State College, Vermont, and she continues work on her bachelor's degree. Married to her high-school sweetheart for over thirty-one years, she and her husband have four grown children. Wanda loves to sing and sings semiprofessionally with a group.

Rosamarie Cruz, MEd, BSN, RN, CSN, grew up in a large family of ten girls and was the only one to go into nursing. Rosamarie is eternally grateful to her mother, who encouraged her to become a nurse. With a master's degree from Cambridge College in Massachusetts, Rosamarie also has earned certifications in basic life support and pediatric advanced life support. Rosamarie loves to spend her free time with her two daughters and her sisters and their families, who all enjoy the beach.

Patricia A. DeLorenze, LPN, pursued all of her education from primary school through nursing school in the town of New Britain, Connecticut. At the end of nursing school in the 1970s, Patricia was given the Student of the Year Award. Her first job following graduation was to care for a newborn, and she has spent much of her nursing career in pediatrics. Patricia has taught first aid and CPR to a variety of student groups, ranging from Girl Scouts to physicians. Her husband, Bob, and she enjoy the outdoors where they live.

Janne M. DeMarco, MS, BS, RN, LPN, CSN, has worked in a psychiatric hospital, in labor and delivery, and in adolescent health; she has taught school nursing at Caldwell College in New Jersey and lectured in various school districts on disasters, such as environmental and school shootings. In 2001, Janne received her master's degree in healthcare management from St. Elizabeth's College in New Jersey. Married to her high-school sweetheart for thirty-three years, she and her husband have three adult children, and they like to travel and babysit for their grandson, Jake. Janne enjoys volunteer work with the students at her high school, working with Bailey, their therapy dog, and in her "spare time" loves reading and gardening.

Julia A. Derouen, MEd, NCC, LPCA, double-majored in psychology and art as an undergraduate at the State University of New York at Geneseo. In 2006, she earned her master's degree in school counseling at Western Carolina University, North Carolina, and she has provided treatment and counseling in substance abuse. Julia has also volunteered for a number of years as an emergency medical technician. To lessen stress, Julia delves into the lost art of black and white photography, as well as drawing and painting.

Wendy Doremus, MS, RN, NP-BC, followed her passion in the area of public health by earning a master's degree in nursing from Pace University, New York. She is certified as a school nurse in the states of New Jersey, Illinois, and Massachusetts. Wendy recently moved to Puerto Rico and is exploring public health care there. She and her husband, Mike, are proud of their four grown children and spend time with them at the ocean whenever possible.

Tamara Dorsett, BSN, RN, earned bachelor's degrees in both elementary education and nursing from Wichita State University, Kansas. In addition to her career in school nursing, she served as an emergency room nurse for ten years. With her husband, William, she has three sons and a wonderful granddaughter, Madison. Her hobbies include swimming, diving, camping, and gardening.

Nina R. Fekaris, MS, BSN, RN, NCSN, garnered the title of Oregon School Nurse of the Year for the 2008–2009 school year. She also served as president of the Oregon School Nurses Association from 2004 to 2007. Nina obtained her master's degree in science from Central Missouri State University. Married to her best friend from high school, George, for twenty-nine years, she is the proud mother of two daughters. Nina also enjoys quilting and cooking.

Laurie Feldkamp, BSN, RN, besides being a school nurse, has nursing experience in the areas of pediatrics, home health care, ambulatory care, and public health care. Laurie recently began to volunteer in a free clinic for the uninsured. She and her husband, Doug, have four grown children and enjoy traveling to visit them. Laurie is a graduate of the University of Michigan.

Laura D. Fell, BSN, RN, worked as a substitute school nurse for twelve years before she began working full-time as a nurse in her school. She also has worked in the hospital setting in orthopedics, cardiac intermediary care, and the newborn nursery. Laura graduated from Northeastern University, Massachusetts with a bachelor's of science in nursing. She has three daughters and a son with her husband, Brian, and likes to camp, hike, and travel.

Barbara L. Filer, BSN, RN, CSN, received her bachelor's of science from the University of Pennsylvania in 1977. She is continuing with master's level course work. She and her husband, Carl, have a grown daughter and plan to travel more in the near future.

Elizabeth (Betty) Fitzpatrick, MS, SNP, RN, graduated from a diploma school in her pursuit to become a registered nurse and then went on to earn certifications as a school nurse practitioner, a hospice and palliative care nurse, and even as a school principal. Semiretired now, Elizabeth continues in hospice work and as a consulting nurse and balances this work with bicycling, reading, and time with her three adult children and grandson.

Phyllis Gentry, RN, lives on a farm with her husband of over thirty-nine years, Danny. The couple enjoys showing beef cattle as well as spending time with their five grandchildren. Phyllis is currently the president of the Kentucky School Nurses Association. Her special interest is health education, and thirteen years ago Phyllis started "Building Blocks," a school club for pregnant and parenting teenagers.

Robin Halemeyer, BSN, RN, CSN, is finishing her master's degree in nursing from McKendree University, Illinois where she also obtained her undergraduate degree. An active member of the Illinois Association of School Nurses as well as the National Association of School Nurses, Robin serves as a nominating committee officer to the latter. Along with her husband, Kevin, and teenage daughter, Hayley, Robin lives in the country, where the family black Labs and cats like to roam.

Kathleen M. Halkins, BSN, RN, recently completed her master's degree in school health at Eastern University, Pennsylvania. Kathleen serves as department chair for the Bethlehem Area School District health Services Department and is the school nurse at Liberty High School. Happily married to her husband, Jim, she is the proud mother of four children and one grandchild, Tanner. Kathleen is a runner and also loves to do counted cross-stitch.

Ruthann Hatt, BSN, RN, a veteran school nurse of over fourteen years, graduated from Northeastern University, Massachusetts. Her career in nursing has spanned many areas of specialty, including the operating room, surgery, geriatrics, and visiting nursing. Ruthann feels that school nursing has tapped every nursing, communication, and counseling skill she has acquired.

Marilyn L. Hebert, BS, RN, was a diploma graduate from the Butterworth Hospital School of Nursing in 1972 and went on to obtain her bachelor's degree from Western Michigan University. In 2009, Marilyn was named Michigan School Nurse of the year. Marilyn has been married to her high-school sweetheart for over thirty-seven years. An outdoorswoman, Marilyn enjoys horseback riding, gardening, and boating.

Marcia Howard, BSN, RN, PHN, has cared for all age levels from preschool through grade twelve in her over twenty-five years of school nursing. A diploma school graduate, she earned her bachelor's from Montana State University and has garnered certifications in various areas, including public health nursing, trauma nursing, and social work. Marcia and her husband like to learn about new cultures and people by way of travel in their motor home.

Tracy Jones, RN, graduated from East Arkansas Community College with a degree in nursing. A single parent, Tracy balances her work in a rural elementary school with quality time with her two young daughters, Jessie Elizabeth and Katie Raegan.

Jean Anne Kamrath, MSFL, BSN, RN, has over twenty years of experience in school nursing. She and her husband of thirty-six years farm and raise cattle. Jean was Nebraska School Nurse of the Year in 2008. She was also given an award for her volunteer work in her "Closet Extravaganza" project, in which dresses were donated to girls who otherwise could not afford to attend their prom.

Sharon L. King, RN, NCSN, obtained an associate's degree in technical nursing from the University of Vermont. Multitalented, she also studied art education and fine arts. Sharon obtained certification as a National Certified School Nurse in 2003. With over nine years of school nursing experience, Sharon also dabbles in art projects, ranging from ceramic animal whistles to ocarinas.

Sunny Kirkham, RN, has worked as a school nurse for over a decade. She is pursuing a course of study with Long Ridge Writers Group. Sunny has been published in *Stepping Stones*, an anthology by writers in Georgia. A student of many topics, Sunny delves into history, dog therapy, and the Bible.

Phyllis E. Kobayashi, School Health Aide, resides in Hawaii where she, her husband, and three sons enjoy the beach. Phyllis has survived more than her share of personal tragedy, including the losses of her first husband to cancer, her eight-year-old daughter to cortical cerebral atrophy, and her father to congestive heart failure. Having witnessed her loved ones' struggles with so many health challenges, Phyllis chose to become a school health aide and offers enduring strength and a balanced view to the children and families she serves.

Donna C. Maginness, BSN, RN, has worked as a school nurse for over seventeen years; she is thankful for opportunities to share hope with kids who may not have had much support in their lives. Donna's previous experience includes work as a pediatric, maternity, and home health nurse. She and her husband, Steve, are proud of their grown children and two granddaughters, Aubrielle and Savannah.

Patricia Marsh-Thorell, BSN, RN, is retired after a twenty-six-year career in school nursing. Patricia loved her job in an elementary school, and she now stays active with dancing, skiing, and fly-fishing.

Vici McClure, BSN, RN, a seasoned school nurse, graduated from the University of Texas at Brownsville. In her current position in an alternative school for pregnant and parenting teenage mothers, Vici brings her clinical experience as a birth educator, lay midwife, and maternal child health nurse. She finds great reward in seeing her students mature, graduate, and even go on to college.

Kayla Mohling, BSN, RN, received her bachelor's of science degree in nursing from South Dakota State University. When not providing care for her students in an urban elementary school, Kayla manages her own shrubbery trimming business. Kayla finds that the nursing instinct in her has led her to adopt homeless pets, and she has three dogs and two cats. Kayla enjoys her three grown children when they come to visit, and her favorite past time is riding her horse, Jozee.

Robert D. Naugle, AND, BFA, is a graduate of southeastern Ohio's Rio Grande College. He also has a bachelor of fine arts degree from Savannah College of Art and Design. In addition to being a school nurse, Robert is a freelance illustrator, with four children's books ready to publish. Robert and his wife, Sheryl, have a young son, Harrison, of whom "Rosie the dog must continuously mask her jealousy."

Mary A. O'Neill, MA, RN, CSN, is retired from twenty-five years in school nursing. In 1948, Mary obtained her registered nursing certification from St. Joseph's School of Nursing in Paterson, New Jersey. Mary went on to obtain her master's degree from Seton Hall University, New Jersey. She and her husband, John, raised nine children. Mary is a thirty-two-year member of the National Nurses Study of Harvard University. The primary focus of this research project is to investigate the potential long-term consequences of the use of oral contraceptives. Mary also volunteers as a Community Emergency Response Team member in her community.

Julie Parker, RN, obtained her bachelor's degree from California State University, Chico. In her work as a school nurse in a large district, Julie travels to multiple school sites each day. She and her husband, Ryan, have three beautiful children, Maddison, Emmett, and Everest. Maddison was recently granted a wish from the Make-a-Wish Foundation, and the family spent a week in Kenya living with giraffes.

Dorothy Patrock, MS, RN, SANE-A, has a master's degree in psychiatric nursing and utilized this in her previous work as a sexual assault examiner. Dorothy is a single mother of two beautiful daughters, both adopted from China. Dorothy regularly reminds herself that with the investments she makes daily in the lives of children, she can never go broke.

Laura Petrowich, BSN, RN, considers the school where she works to be in a rural setting "by Lower 48 standards." Laura feels it is a privilege to work at the same school attended by her children, Maverick and Sarah. A graduate of Southeast Missouri State University, Laura and her family enjoy summer vacations in Ninilchik, Alaska, where they hunt for razor clams under the midnight sun.

Carol Ray, LPN, attended and became a licensed practical nurse through her work at South Central Michigan School of Nursing. She and her son, Johnny, live in a small rural community, where they relax by playing catch with their Labrador, Gracy.

Gloria Jean Reynolds, BSN, RN, CSN, earned her bachelor's degree from Webster University in St. Louis, Missouri. Gloria has worked as a school nurse for over twelve years. She and her husband of thirty-nine years, Edgar Ray, enjoy camping with their children, grandchildren, and long-haired Chihuahua, Snickers.

Jeanmarie Ringwood, MA, RN, CSN, after ten years of school nursing, is thankful that she made the choice to enter this field because she learns on a daily basis from her patients, students, families, and coworkers. To broaden her skills, she obtained a master's in health education from Montclair University, New Jersey. In her free time, she enjoys exercise and spending time with her husband and their three children.

Lori E. Robson, BSN, RN, CSN, began her career as a cardiac nurse but found her niche in school nursing. She graduated from Seton Hall University and obtained her school nurse certification at Caldwell College in New Jersey. Lori is an avid country music fan and also considers shopping as "sport."

Shirley Rodriguez, BSN, RN, CSNP, studied nursing at various colleges: San Bernardino Valley College in California, the University of Colorado, and the University of Phoenix, where she earned her bachelor's degree. She was the president of the School Nurses Organization of Arizona and a vice president of the National Association of School Nurses. She has participated on many local, state, and national boards and committees that aim to impact health, nursing, and the welfare of children. Shirley and her husband have two married children and two wonderful grandchildren, who attend the school where Shirley works.

Laurie Rufolo, MSN, RN, works as a school nurse in an urban setting. She received her master's degree from Wagner College in Staten Island, New York and earned her school nurse certification from Seton Hall University, New Jersey. Laurie and her husband volunteer in Scouting, as her husband and two sons are Eagle Scouts. Currently, Laurie is engaged in a special school nursing project, in which she works with academically failing students as they reinvent themselves as capable students.

Carol Ann Scalgione, RN, graduated from the Rutgers University College of Nursing, New Jersey. She is deeply grateful for the journey of her nursing career of over thirty-one years. She and her husband, Richard, enjoy downtime with their two sons. Their dog, Anna, and cat, Lily Ann, complete the family unit.

Melanie Sharpton, RN, divides her time between working in a rural high school and enjoying home life with her husband and two daughters, Jessica and Hannah. During the hot summer days, the family cools off by boating and tubing on the lake.

Tamara J. Smylie, BS, RN, NCSN, a school nurse, obtained National School Nurse Certification in 2007. She and her husband are active in their church and love to backpack and fish in the mountains. Tamara feels that her four children have made her a better nurse.

Alexis J. Strickland, RN, has been tested by over twenty-seven years of experience in school nursing. Her future plans include becoming an advocate for nursing home residents. Alexis and her husband, Ken, had two sons. Their youngest boy died at age eighteen, and Alexis attributes her ability to cope to her deep faith and the support of her family. Alexis and Ken enjoy camping and day trips with their ten grandchildren.

Renie Sullivan, MEd, BSN, RN, graduated with a master's in health education from Rhode Island College. Renie juggles work in an elementary school with her night jobs as a hospital administrative coordinator and an IV therapy nurse. This work in the hospital helps Renie to stay current in the field. In her limited spare time, Renie loves riding in her 1968 Mustang convertible, which was a thirtieth anniversary gift from her husband.

Candi Thomas, BSN, RN, has a busy life in a rural community, where she works as a school nurse for students in preschool through high school and is also a mother to her two toddlers, Skyler and Kynzi. Someday, when her children are a bit older, Candi plans to return to nursing in labor and delivery.

Verna Thompson, BSN, RN, previously worked as a head nurse on a surgery floor in a medical center. She stayed home to have and care for her three children for ten years before returning to nursing. Verna feels blessed that she has been in school nursing for the past seven years. When not at school or being Mom, Verna helps her husband with their dairy farm and enjoys working with youth at her church and in the local Scout troop.

Heidi Toth, MS, MSN, RN, CIC, has garnered many degrees and certifications, with the most recent being a master's in health sciences at New Jersey City University, as well as additional studies in educational supervision at Kean University. As an adjunct professor at New Jersey City University and Monmouth University, Heidi imparted clinical experience as well as her preschool through high school nursing expertise to her students. Recognized by numerous professional organizations, Heidi was the New Jersey State School Nurse of the Year in 2007–2008. An accomplished researcher, Heidi published a chapter on Lyme disease in the 2005 edition of *Individualized Health Care Plans for the School Nurse* by Sunrise Press. She has presented talks on "Efficacy of a Peer-to-Peer Education Program Regarding Substance Abuse" and "Stress and Coping in New Jersey School Nurses." Heidi works tirelessly in many volunteer capacities, such as Scout leading, Little League coaching, and contributing to various community organizations.

Patti J. Twaddle, RN, worked in medical and surgery, pediatric, and labor and delivery nursing before becoming a school nurse in a rural school district. She stays very busy with her husband of twenty-one years and their four children. Outside of family life and nursing, her great passion is photography, as she loves freezing time with a camera lens.

Sherri Verdun, BS, RN, CSN, obtained her school nurse certification from National Lewis University in 1998. Previously, she obtained a bachelor's degree in accounting and made a major career change from this field to nursing. A sports enthusiast, she coaches volleyball and enjoys following her four children in their sports activities. Sherri and her husband recently moved their bustling family into a new home that they built themselves.

Domichellei Walker, RN, graduated from Centralia College in Washington with an associate's degree in nursing. Domichellei, who works as a school nurse in a rural area, considers herself to be one of the lucky few who love their job. She and her husband and two children enjoy camping and boating every year.

Ellen Williams, MEd, BSN, RN, received her master's degree from Cambridge College in Boston and is the current treasurer for the New Mexico School Nurse Association. A school nurse for over fourteen years, Ellen has a wide-ranging nursing career that has had roles from pediatrics to a burn unit to the ER. Ellen and her husband's six grown children have spawned ten grandchildren, and they all enjoy family get-togethers. Ellen plays the violin in a community orchestra and also enjoys reading and crossword puzzles.

Beth H. Wipf, BSN, RN, earned her bachelor of science degree in nursing from Georgia University. As a school nurse, Beth has drawn on her experience in pediatric nursing in Kentucky, Ohio, and Arizona. She and her husband parent three active children and enjoy beach activities by their current home